Be Your Own Nutritionist

Be Your Own Nutritionist

RETHINK YOUR RELATIONSHIP WITH FOOD

GEORGE COOPER

SB

Published in 2013 by Short Books

Short Books
3A Exmouth House
Pine Street
EC1R 0JH

10 9 8 7 6 5 4 3 2 1

A CIP catalogue record for this book
is available from the British Library.

ISBN 978-1-78072-156-9

Printed in Great Britain by CPI Group (UK) Ltd.
Croydon, CR0 4YY

Helen

With special thanks to Jamie Richards & Shona Rodger

Go to:
www.george-cooper.co.uk
for more recipes and commentaries and
to sign up for newsletters.

Contents

Introduction

It's a typical day in my Bristol clinic as I start a consultation with a new client. She has been in pain for a long time and nothing that has been recommended to her over the years has seemed to work. Now she is low in confidence and badly in need of an effective route to health.

I explain to her the origin of her illness from scientific and traditional points of view. She is not unusual; her diet – one mainly made up of harmful and addictive foods such as cheap meat products, pastries, crisps, high-fat sandwiches, white factory bread, puddings and sweets – has exacted a steady and destructive toll on her constitution. I tell her that the only way that she is going to get better is by changing her nutritional habits and bringing her daily diet back into balance. My role in the process is initially therapeutic and normally requires medicine, but, once she has regained her health, if she is to continue to be well and happy, she will have to learn to manage her diet according to her changing needs for years to come. She will have to become a food expert; she will have to be her own nutritionist.

My client is one of millions of modern Britons who are suffering from diet-induced disease, a shocking diagnosis for which there is incontrovertible proof.

Over recent years, the burden of digestive disease in Britain has increased – some ten years ago malnutrition was thought to cost the UK in excess of £7.3bn a year,[1] and that figure has steadily risen to over £16bn. Indeed, all populations that adopt the same pattern of eating are suffering digestively. People throughout the developed world are fatter, becoming increasingly diabetic and suffering near epidemic levels of cancer, heart attacks and strokes.

If the case for us all to be our own nutritionists is compelling, the problem is that, generally speaking, we simply don't seem to have the tools to create and sustain a healthy diet as a nutritionist does. There are so many different ideas of what healthy foods are, how and when to eat them and such a profusion of different dietary theories that those who *do* want to eat healthily are baffled from the outset.

Hence this book, in which I aim to address this confusion head-on, and to arm readers with exactly the sort of tools they need to understand and fulfil their own nutritional needs. It is my strong belief that, after years of lassitude in this area, we need – collectively – to establish a clear sense of nutritional direction. We need to develop a new relationship with what we eat, a genuinely *healthy* diet that is clearly understood and that will sit comfortably within our mainstream culture.

And, guess what? The information that is required to construct such a diet is nothing new or fancy; *everything that we need to know can already be found within contemporary science and tradition*. It just has to be put together in a way that is relevant and adaptable. Read on!

---

1 Elia M, Stratton R, Russell C, Green C, Pan F (2005). The cost of disease-related malnutrition in the UK: considerations for the use of oral nutritional supplements (ONS) in adults. *BAPEN New Health Economic Report*. Worcestershire BAPEN,

My diet plan is based on personal experience – the result of a journey I embarked upon some time ago, prompted by long-term illness and a gradual and relentless deterioration of my own health.

I started out – and grew up – a sickly child: snotty, weak and occasionally entertaining in my puny efforts at jumping, throwing and brawling. Entertaining to my older brothers at least. And I'm afraid to say that for eighteen long years I conspicuously failed to get one over on my brothers as I muddled through the rough-and-tumble of childhood and adolescence.

Things got really bad when, as a student, I spent a couple of months in Indonesia. I caught *Giardia* and started to vomit. And vomit. In fact, I vomited unremittingly up to three times a day, every day for eighteen months.

The impact on my health was grim and relentless. My weight plummeted dangerously and malnourishment set in. I went to my GP who sent me to a physician who recommended a combination of drugs. When these didn't work I took them again, with no improvement. I then took a different set of drugs. Again, with no improvement. In fact, over eighteen months I took nine different sets of drugs – all to no avail – and I just kept on vomiting. My instinct was that I didn't want to keep taking drugs, especially if they didn't actually help. This instinct was more than vindicated when I discovered that one of the drugs I had been taking is highly addictive, two of them actually have vomiting listed as a side effect (!) and another has since been banned for its destructive effect on heart health.

So I consulted a stomach surgeon and eventually

followed his advice to go under the knife. In January 1995 I had a fundoplication, a procedure that places a muscular restriction around the top of the stomach to make vomiting impossible. I woke from the anaesthetic with a sneeze, rendered somewhat excruciating by the 22 stitches in my abdomen. I also became an insomniac, possibly due to the trauma of the surgery, possibly because my left lung had collapsed during the surgery, or possibly due to the anaesthetic drugs; possibly due to all three. And I started to retch and continued to retch.

This was the end of the road for me and conventional medicine. I had exhausted all ideas – drugs, surgery and various practitioners' frankly risible dietary advice – and emerged sick, in pain, sleep-deprived and with a surgically altered stomach.

It was time to start finding out answers myself, and so I turned to the alternatives and began to read up on diet in particular.

There were a few options available in those days: yoga, homeopathy, hypnosis, medical herbalism, spiritual acupuncture, detox therapy. But the only one that cut the mustard with me was traditional Chinese medicine, an ancient, complex and elegant holistic system of acupuncture, herbalism, dietary and exercise therapy, and massage.

Whereas conventional medicine had no definitions for my illness and therefore could not provide appropriately directed and effective treatment, Chinese medicine quickly gave me a specific diagnosis for my condition, with specific and detailed solutions. My sickness, it turned out, was caused by a rather dramatic combination of anxiety and a weak stomach. In the end the analysis was simple: some people get butterflies when they're nervous; they experience nausea; they throw up. I was anxious and nervous all the time and threw up all the time! Because my stomach was weak, the nerves could easily overpower it and disrupt its harmonious function.

Understanding the nature of my condition was a huge breakthrough. From then on, I resolved to heal myself. I trained in natural medicine, developing a profound sense of illness and therapeutics along the way and ending up with a clinical career by default. That clinical career has been instrumental in the development of the ideas for dietary health I set out in this book, as I have transmitted my discoveries to my clients to ameliorate their own health issues. This diet (based on what I have found to be the five key factors for dietary health: climate, gut function, emotion, flavour analysis and food type) now underpins my own health and the health of thousands of my clients and their families. If you follow it, you too will be well on your way to becoming your own nutritionist.

***

When it comes to diets for health, nothing quite compares to the traditional Chinese approach. This is supported by numerous and extremely detailed anthropological, epidemiological and nutritional studies. Traditional Chinese nutrition underpins the diet of the healthiest and longest-living populations in the world: those of Japan, Hong Kong and Singapore. And not only is this approach remarkably healthy, it is also truly versatile. It can be adapted to all climates (which, as you will learn, have a profound effect on our health and the food we should eat), seasons, lifestyles, foods and illnesses in the world.

For years, however, I struggled to relate the logic of the traditional Chinese approach to our British culture. Chinese nutrition might be versatile, I thought, but was it not just a bit too exotic? How would my British clients relate to it? And then I came upon a series of academic papers detailing another exceptionally healthy diet, one based on many of the same principles, but, interestingly, developed much closer to home – the mid-Victorian working-class diet.[2] [3]

The papers describing this phenomenal British diet – the healthiest one, incidentally, that this country has ever known – were of particular interest to me because, as I read them, it became evident that it shared extensive similarities with the Chinese-based diet that I had constructed. So why had it been lost to us? The Chinese had retained their connection with their dietary past. In Britain, and much of the developed world, however, we seemed to have lost touch with our roots altogether. As the authors of the papers, Drs Clayton and Rowbotham, say: "The inescapable message is that the brief dietary advances of the mid-Victorian period have been lost to us... in our rush to embrace the pharmaceutical model of healthcare (which largely springs from the success of the early antibiotics), we have allowed the nutritional wisdom of the mid-Victorian era to be squandered."

Let's start with some of those striking similarities between the mid-Victorian diet and my own Chinese-based one. Both:

- use foods in relation to variations in digestibility, climate, season, lifestyle, stage of life, emotion and disease

2   Clayton P & Rowbotham J (2009). How the Mid-Victorians Worked, Ate and Died. *Intern. Journal Environ. Res. Public Health*, 6: 1235-53
3   Clayton P & Rowbotham J (2008). An unsuitable and degraded diet? Public health lessons from the mid-Victorian working-class diet. Parts 1,2 & 3, *Journal Royal Society of Medicine*

- are diagnostic in nature and adaptable for individual cases
- are extremely diverse
- are packed with vegetables, nuts, seeds and fruit
- put a special emphasis on rich foods like fish, animal and plant fats as an adaptation to cold and damp climate, and place these in the context of aromatic, warm, cooked and hearty dishes to enhance digestibility
- use fermented foods, strongly flavoured herbs, spices and condiments extensively
- rely on regular consumption of medicinal foods such as offal, shellfish, walnuts, chestnuts and certain herbs and spices to extend life and sustain health.

The logic of the Chinese and Japanese diet is entirely conscious, of course. It is extensively detailed in a substantial literature, and there is an explicable, health-based reason for every aspect of it, wherever it is being applied.

For the mid-Victorian working class, by contrast, there is no way – due in large part to illiteracy – that we can know that every health-enhancing aspect of their diet was deliberate rather than a happy accident. I will, however, endeavour to demonstrate that in many specific cases they knew exactly what they were doing.

In this book, I will provide an effective guide to recovering the wisdom of our forebears by referring to other major traditions that *have* survived into modern times, principally those from China and Japan. You can therefore use the book as a culturally relevant foundation to develop your food expertise in relation to the five major factors that should determine your diet: climate, emotion, the properties and flavours of foods, and the subtleties of digestive function. Get to grips with these relationships and you are well on your way to becoming your own nutritionist.

My intention is that *Be Your Own Nutritionist* has a genuine impact on your health and appreciation of food – for the rest of your lives. Enjoy the book – and, who knows, in time, we British might just gain a reputation as a healthy bunch after all!

1.

The Golden Age of British Diet

Today, we are relatively distant from our food. While there are different approaches to food analysis and classification, both scientific and traditional, none of them hold a steady, consistent place in our culture. In fact, there seems to be a huge amount of doubt and misunderstanding around what we eat.

Our practical day-to-day relationship with nutrition seems to have suffered too. We tend not to think about how climate impacts on our health and food. Similarly, we pay little attention to how we might change our diet to alleviate the symptoms caused by our emotions. And, once food is eaten, there is virtually no cultural awareness of how our digestion works and the pivotal role of digestive processes in determining our well-being.

To be your own nutritionist, you need to understand these things. Most Chinese and Japanese, for example, *are* their own nutritionists, as their dietary culture – with its long history and deep and subtle analysis of food – is strong. And this was once also the case in Britain.

So let's take a look back at our dietary history; there we

will find the clues that show us why those five factors – emotion, climate, digestive function and food flavour and type – are so fundamental to health.

Origins

The needs of modern man are not unique. Despite the great changes that our societies have undergone in recent years, many of the factors that we have to take into account when it comes to our health and diet have always affected us, from the very beginning of the evolution of man.

Throughout human history, our quality of life, our longevity and, in many cases, our survival, have depended on our ability to adapt to varying circumstances, and on our having a profound understanding of not just ecology – plants, animals, fungi and micro-organisms – but also of the changing seasons, shifting weather patterns and unique topographies, and how they relate to food availability and well-being. In other words, our ancestors have always needed to be nutritionists with a sophisticated appreciation of their own changing needs.

***

So how did the modern human diet evolve? The two major vectors for the development of diet in the ancient world were trade and religion. As a by-product of the dissemination of goods and beliefs, ideas and foods were constantly exchanged; by Arab traders along the Silk Route, by European travellers and diplomats such as Marco Polo and by Christian and Buddhist missionaries. With the development of hieroglyphs and writing, this essential dietary knowledge came to be recorded. Indeed, the historical exchange of ideas was so fluid that it is documented that an idea could cross the world in under two years. This cross-fertilisation led to striking similarities in the dietary philosophies evolving throughout the ancient world.

Our Western dietary culture, therefore, grew as much as anything from Eastern roots. In the sixteenth and seventeenth centuries dietary medicine in the West reached its zenith – and many of the theories at this time were similar to those in China and Japan.

In this epoch, the ability to eat a consistently sustaining diet was difficult for the urban and rural poor, but the nobility did not have this problem. And, since this diet was recorded, it is possible to learn from its insights and compare it to the healthy modern-day dietary traditions of places such as Japan and Hong Kong (first and second respectively in the global life expectancy rankings).

The similarities are extraordinary:

- *Cooking* was seen as an extension of the digestive process itself, a vital process designed to break down the structure of the food so that, once it was eaten, it could be easily absorbed.
- *Appetite* was also considered important, with meals starting with spiced wines, drinks and sweets using ingredients such as ginger, caraway, anise, fennel and cumin: products that were valued as appetisers. (In China and Japan today, similar spices are used at the beginning of a meal to encourage *kai wei* or "open stomach").
- Foods were also *classified according to their affect on the body once they had been eaten*, from "cooling" to "heating" and from "drying" to "moistening". This

reflects the Eastern traditional view of foods having *yin* or *yang* properties. Such classification of foods was, and is, very useful. Today in the hot, humid summers typical of Hong Kong, cooling and bitter drying foods are considered very important.

• Most notably, another classification of foods in medieval times was based on *digestibility*, with the most digestible foods in a meal prioritised over the least digestible. Thus, meals would start with fruit dishes followed by a wide range of cooked vegetables, herbs, soups, broths and light meats such as chicken and rabbit. Only then would richer foods be considered, such as pork, beef and nuts. Hard cheeses were preferred to soft, as these were aged and easier to digest, and bitter, sweet and aromatic digestives would finish a meal.

We see exactly the same principles in traditional Asian cuisine, where a meal is not considered balanced unless it is digestible – the two key principles of digestibility being how a dish is cooked and how its flavours are combined (principles which are expanded on later in this book).

The healthiest Britons ever

What the historical record shows us is that parts of British society always had the knowledge and resources to eat healthily, with dietary theories and practices that compare favourably with the healthiest and longest-living populations in the world today. Indeed, it is likely that such knowledge was more widespread than historians might have given our ancestors credit for. For example, in rural areas, there has long been a tradition of "Herb Wives". These women harboured and transmitted medicinal insights; but because they were not literate, much of their knowledge was never recorded and therefore is not recognised today. To hard-working peasants, however, such knowledge meant the difference between life and death.

What we do know is that the healthiest period in British history, when society had the most nutritional tools at its disposal, was the mid-Victorian era. During this period, a brief, but significant, Golden Age of British Diet was ushered in.

It all began with improvements to agriculture in the late seventeenth century. These peaked in the mid-nineteenth century when a change to the system of crop rotation raised arable output and improved animal husbandry. This involved using crops like turnips and swede that have the ability to replenish the soil and can be used to fatten livestock over winter. In addition, crucially, in 1845 the Corn Laws were repealed, ensuring access to cheap food for all, including the urban masses. It was then down to the newly built railways to get that food into the cities where it was needed, a function that was performed so effectively that malnutrition and starvation rates at that time matched rather than exceeded those of today's era of cheap and abundant food.

The impact of these changes on the nation's health was dramatic. Mid-Victorians became the toughest – and healthiest – Britons ever, and in this context I am referring to the working class, who made up 75% of the population. It is true that during this period a lot of young children died due to poor understanding and treatment of infectious diseases and primitive perinatal techniques. Similarly many women died in and around childbirth, including the famous

Mrs Beeton. However, once these factors are accounted for, statistics from 1850 to 1875 show that working-class men and women outlived today's British working class and had more or less the same average life expectancy. This is amazing when you think that, in the absence of family planning, mid-Victorian women had to cope with up to 30 years of successive pregnancies and births and the working conditions were so much harsher.

While these figures are impressive in themselves, it is also notable that in the absence of modern drugs, central heating, sanitation, surgery, pensions and other conveniences, the mid-Victorians were also much *healthier* than us. They were ten times less likely to experience degenerative disease such as heart attacks, strokes and cancers. Consequently, they would live a vibrant life and die very quickly from infectious disease or trauma at the end of it.

Today, by contrast, our final years are characterised by suffering, with men typically spending their last eight years, and women their last ten, in increasing medical dependency. Much of modern healthcare is about keeping us alive in a degraded state rather than building and maintaining health in the first place. It often seems to me that in modern Britain we operate a National *Disease* Service rather than a National Health Service.

The vitality of the mid-Victorians is illustrated by their sheer physical strength and high activity levels. They could eat more than twice as many calories as we do today, with negligible associated obesity. For a start, low-paid workers often walked up to six miles a day. Women would spend all day on their feet in factories before heading home to the chores, which seemed to involve hours of scrubbing. Single women were often employed as live-in domestic help, scrubbing and lugging coal and water.

Many men worked as hard, managing 55 to 75 hours of work-related physical activity a week before popping out for a bit of market gardening or a game of football (something of a rough sport in those days compared with today's tempered version). At the top end of the scale, there were the "navigators", the men who built the railways and expended 5000 calories a day, while brick makers produced 1000 bricks an hour during a 58-hour week. One sprightly fellow is recorded to have made 986,091 bricks in five months! Manly stuff.

So, what is the diet that sustained these amazing people? Crucially, it was organically produced (there was nothing else), it was seasonal, local, thrifty and diverse; everything that today's typical diet isn't.

Truly fresh fruit and vegetables

The mid-Victorians ate huge amounts of onions, watercress, leeks, carrots and turnips, as well as Jerusalem artichokes, all of which are easily home grown. Cabbage and broccoli were cheap and widely available and beans and peas were eaten fresh during summer and early autumn. Dried beans and other pulses were available all year round and were a key staple. Dried fruit was also eaten throughout the year, while classic British varieties, including apples, cherries, gooseberries, plums and greengages, were consumed fresh and in season.

Nuts

Hazelnuts, walnuts and chestnuts were popular and were widely available as they could be gathered from hedgerows, a great seasonal ritual that coincided with school holidays;

sadly, virtually all of this tradition is lost to us as a result of modern agriculture and our predominantly urban lifestyles.

Making the most of fish and meat

Another contrast with modern times was the preparation of fish; herring in particular. It was eaten whole, including the highly nutritious heads and roes, and was also dried, pickled, jellied and salted for year-round use, as were sprats, eels, oysters, mussels, cockles and whelks. Cod, haddock and John Dory were eaten too. Everyone ate fish and meat, if they could afford it. The dietary absence of meat was rare and generally a sign of extreme poverty, and as with fish, nothing was wasted. All the offal was eaten – with relish, I might add – and the bones were used for stocks and broths. The animal fat was also treasured, with dripping used as the working man's "butter". Beyond this, it was common to have a couple of chickens in the back yard, turning kitchen scraps back into fresh food in the form of eggs.

This "use everything" approach has clear benefits for health. Offal, such as liver, kidneys, sweetbreads and tongue, is demonstrably more rich, and varied, in nutrients than the usual musculoskeletal meat that we tend to focus on today.[4]

Cheap food

The cheapness of many of these foods combined with thrift and the ability to grow their own produce meant that for

---

4   McCance RA, Widdowson EM (2006). *The Composition of Foods*. 6th Edition. London: Food Standards Agency

the mid-Victorian working class, money for onions, cherries, apples, bones, dripping, offal and meat scraps was not typically included in household budgets. They were so easy to obtain. This has led some modern historians to draw false conclusions about the Victorian era; the fact that homegrown foods were not accounted for in budgets made them believe that they weren't eaten at all!

Nothing could be further from the truth. Food was abundant and the working class were predominantly well fed. Average consumption figures from 1851 bear this out: eight pounds of pears per person per annum compared with three now; double the amount of soft fruit and more than five times the amount of dried fruit compared to today. For vegetables, the average mid-Victorian Londoner ate nearly three times as many onions, eighteen times more turnips and swedes and more than three times as many cabbages.[5]

They ended up with a weekly menu that might have looked something like this:

Sunday Lunch
A joint
[normally boiled – rather than roasted – which created a delicious broth, dispersed the richness of the meat, minimising the loss of nutrients and reducing the formation of carcinogenic chemicals caused by cooking]

Monday
Porridge or stoneground bread with leftovers
or cold meat with salad greens, bread and pickles

---

5   Bryson B (2011). *At Home*. London: Black Swan

Tuesday
Meat leftovers from Sunday, hashed or spiced
[The bones provided stock for soup with vegetables and pulses]

Wednesday and Thursday
Suet crusts and gravy
with vegetables or salad greens

Rice, beans and other pulses
with seasonal nuts and vegetables
*[Meat was normally off the menu for the poorest
as pay day was Friday!]*

A steamed meat suet pudding
[for the wealthier workers]

Friday
Fish
or fish head soup
[for the poorest]

Saturday
Chops, steak
or stewed offal
[for the poorest]
*

Plenty of seasonal nuts, veg and fruit

Hearty, nourishing stuff, and, incredibly, once we account for the obviously toxic food adulterants of this era, such as arsenic compounds, many of the other substances that were unscrupulously added to food were actually health enhancing. This included hawthorn, which was added to pad out tea and coriander which was put into beer. Meanwhile, "contaminant" yeasts that grew on bread and unfiltered beer produced health-promoting beta glucans; a happy accident that can't occur today, due to the over-refinement of ingredients and zealous sanitisation of production environments.

So, the mid-Victorian diet was the healthiest that Britain has ever seen. Its diversity and scope meant that it was extremely adaptable for changing circumstances such as climate and food availability – a key requirement for nutritionists. It was also nutritionally dense, essential for low morbidity and high longevity. These are fundamental characteristics that are shared by today's healthiest diets, like that of Japan. (For a long time now, the Japanese have been the longest-living people in the world, closely followed by the residents of Hong Kong, a fact backed up by a 25-year study of the Okinawans,[6] the longest-living and healthiest of the Japanese, and therefore of all humankind.)

These characteristics are also shared by the diet in parts of the Mediterranean. The Mediterranean diet, as we know, is much studied and credited in modern times with being the major contributor to the relatively low levels of obesity and heart disease, in southern European countries like southern France, Italy, Cyprus and Spain. In terms of lifestyle and approaches to food we can learn a lot from these healthy cultures – they form a bridge to recreating our own.

First, though, we should look in detail at the Golden Age of British Diet of 150 years ago and assess how it relates to our physiology and modern lifestyles, how we might embellish it with the best of today's traditional diets, and relearn what it is to eat truly healthily.

---

6   see Wilcox B, Wilcox D & Suzuki M (2001) The Okinawa Program, New York, Three Rivers Press

The French paradox

The traditional French diet has led to the "French Paradox": that they are remarkably healthy despite high levels fat in their food. This is only a paradox in modern terms, of course. The mid-Victorians ably demonstrated that it's not how much fat you eat, but the type of fat, how you eat it and how much you exercise that matter.

2.

What Went Wrong with Modern Diets

Remember how I said that the Golden Age of British diet was so brief? A mere 25 years, from 1850 to 1875. After this, the British diet started to change, with catastrophic health consequences. In 1874 Gladstone abolished sugar tax; sugar became cheap and sugary processed foods were mass-produced, mass-marketed and consumed in extraordinary quantities. The late Victorians' teeth rotted and fell out. They could no longer eat the fibrous fruit, vegetables and nuts enjoyed by their parents. Fresh-meat consumption declined as cheaper canned and salted meat was imported from abroad and white flour became the norm for baking.

It is easy to see how hard this hit us. Within two generations, British men went from the navvies who could shovel 20 tonnes of earth a day *each*, to a puny bunch, 50% of whom were rejected as unfit for service in the second Boer war due to malnourishment. The minimum height requirement for the infantry was reduced from 5'6" to a mere 5' and the middle-class officers – whose diet declined much less rapidly – stood a full head higher than their men.

In 1904 the government stepped in to try to remedy the

situation, initiating the provision of school meals for working-class children. But, in general terms, the decline in our diets continued.

In the 1920s the dentist and nutritionist Weston Price toured the world documenting the impact of modern dietary changes. In Britain, he could find only one population that still ate truly traditionally. This was on the Isle of Lewis in the Hebrides. Their diet was based on barley, oats and fish, which they ate whole; a typical dish being baked cod's head stuffed with chopped liver and oatmeal. The health of these islanders was incredible; they were strong and their teeth had remarkably few dental cavities. By this time, however, the diet in the island's port of Stornoway had changed witht he introduction of sugar and white flour. The result was poor growth among the children and rotten teeth for the townies. It didn't take long for the sugar and white flour to spread across the island too. The demise of the traditional British diet was complete.

The rise and rise of junk food

The sugar and white flour that did for the Victorians has now, in combination with cheap modified fat and excessive salt, come to dominate the "Western Diet". It affects nearly every population in the world, including even the Okinawans, who are losing their healthy lustre because they are adopting modern dietary habits and getting fatter, and dying younger.

The Western Diet transcends class and has undermined and infiltrated nutrition in every layer of society, to the extent that the most health-conscious of us are still exposed to it through hidden salt in shop-bought salads, hidden sugar and salt in breakfast cereals or cheap fat and additives in sandwiches, biscuits, ice cream and cakes. It is likely that, if you don't prepare everything yourself from high quality ingredients, you'll always be exposed to some aspect of the Western Diet.

It is easy enough to see how the Western Diet became ubiquitous. A good starting point is recent research that suggests that eating salt, sugar and cheap fat triggers the same addictive neurological pathways as heroin consumption and withdrawal.[789]. In other words, some ingredients – the types of ingredients that are invariably found in ready meals and junk food snacks – seem to be truly addictive; and as consumers, intentionally or not, we are damaging ourselves by eating them.

One of the methods that junk food manufacturers and retailers use to promote and market their products is to manipulate the language of science. They take a cheap and unhealthy product with a low nutritional value, packed with ingredients that create compulsion like salt and sugar, and then cover the boxes, packets and wrappers with scientific terminology that gives the illusion of health and nutrition.

7   Liedtke W et al. (2011) Relation of addiction genes to hypothalamic gene changes subserving genesis and gratification of a classic instinct, sodium appetite. Proceedings of the National Academy of Sciences www.pnas. org/cgi/doi/10.1073/pnas.1109199108

8   Burger K. & Stice E. (2012) Frequent ice cream consumption is associated with reduced striatal response to receipt of an ice cream–based milkshake. American Journal of Nutrition February 15, doi: 10.3945/ ajcn.111.02700

9   Johnson PM & Kenny PJ (2010) Dopamine D2 receptors in addiction-like reward dysfunction and compulsive eating in obese rats Nature Neuroscience 13 pp635-41

The result is that, more often than not, processed food is mutton dressed as lamb.[10] As consumers of the Western Diet, we compulsively eat nutritionally deficient food, often under the illusion that it is good for us.

Case study

Brenda, 31, was a keen triathlete. She came to me with Chronic Fatigue Syndrome; she was too tired to train and compete and had not had a period for over a year. Her demanding job was also a struggle. I diagnosed her primarily with weak digestion, poor motility and weak blood.

Brenda's main problem was that, as a vegetarian, her diet was nowhere near rich enough to sustain her in her intensive exercise regime and hard job. I got her eating lots of plant fats and lots of eggs. Eggs of all sorts: duck, quail, hen and goose. All these rich foods were combined with sour flavours and aromatic herbs and spices to improve digestibility. Fats were often eaten in a dressing. She also had acupuncture to improve digestive efficiency and herbal tonics for blood and digestion.

Brenda's energy levels improved more or less immediately. Three months later her periods returned; four months later she could exercise again and she was able to compete in the next triathlon season.

---

10 A number of books and articles have been written on food corporations and the junk food industry – it is an extensive subject. Michael Pollan's *In Defence of Food* is a good starting point

Banish the fads

In recent decades many people have turned to diets other than the Western Diet in an attempt to undo its harm, and in particular to lose weight. These alternative diets – or rather, fad diets – ostensibly exist to promote health and weight loss, but in reality they share many of the failings of the Western Diet.

Looking back over the past half-century, we have been offered a steady stream of high-protein, low-protein, high-carb, low-carb, calorie-controlled, eat-what-you-want, blood-type and raw-food diets – all contradicting each other in scientific-sounding ways, despite seeming to have the same goals of weight loss and health enhancement. Not all of these diets can be right in their stated benefits and it's up to us to work out where the dietary value lies, a process that can be bewilderingly complex.

The extraordinary number of fad diets and slimming companies, combined with the tons of "health foods" that are eaten in this country, show that there is a genuine desire to eat healthier foods. And yet, as a nation, under the aegis of scientific progress, we are experiencing more and more food-related illness.

Big business

It isn't difficult to see that this rise in diet-related illness has come about as a result of the machinations of food corporations. They exist to maximise profit for their shareholders – and that means selling more junk food!

Just like any marketplace, a fad diet is as successful as its proponent's ability to sell it, through PR, marketing, and celebrity and media connections. That's why there are so many of them around, in book shops, on the web, TV and other media; lots of people want to cash in on such a big market.

Sometimes, there may be a very genuine motivation behind the selling of a fad diet, because it worked for its originator. They are passionate about the diet because, they say, it solved a health issue or made them feel healthy and vibrant – at least for a certain time. But does that mean that the same diet would work for everyone else? Definitely not.

Not just another fad diet

So is this diet another fad? No, for the simple reason that it is founded in tradition; *our* historical tradition and one which sustained our healthiest-ever population. And it is embellished by other foreign traditions that have kept massive numbers of people in health for centuries. I am not using ideas that have only worked in a very specific context, for individuals or small groups of people, and then generalising them for all people in all circumstances. Nor am I embracing the spin of commercial vested interests. Rather, the ideas behind this diet are ancient *and* modern, tried and tested throughout whole societies in a range of latitudes, terrains, climates and ethnicities. As we learn more about these diets we can begin to adapt their principles to our own needs – to suit us as individuals. So, more than any other, this will be *your* diet.

Case Study

Phil, a male in his mid-thirties, presented with a symptom that I have seen many times in my clinic. He had a pain in his lower right abdomen that radiated down the inside of his right thigh. The docs had checked everything out, his appendix, possible hernias, cancer even, and found "nothing". But the pain persisted. Analysing his symptoms from a traditional perspective, it seemed he had a problem with a sluggish and cramping gut, which also caused the radiating pain down his leg.

Phil's diet wasn't bad, but could be improved. He ate too much raw veg, drank too much booze and, importantly, drank "sugar-free", "diet" fizzy drinks, with their potentially toxic additives. Phil was given some acupuncture and aromatic herbs to stimulate gut movement. He also ate more cooked food, cut down on beer and cut out processed food and drink (mostly!). He's now pain free, and losing weight too.

3.

About Digestion

It was nearly twenty years ago that I found myself with severe stomach disease, and at my wit's end. The medical profession, including some of the most reputable gastro-enterological surgeons and physicians in Bristol, had given me all they had to offer, and my GP had neither the time, nor the training to suggest where to look next. I was experiencing the limitations of one health culture, and was forced to look to others for answers.

Why, you might ask, is the scientific nutritional knowledge of our doctors apparently so limited?

The problem for modern gastroenterological science is the complexity of the human gut, and the breathtaking nutritional diversity of the food that we put in it.

In terms of anatomy an average human adult gut is nine metres long and consists of at least seven different sections. It is serviced by two major secreting organs, and the nerves that supply it weigh the same as the brain and the spinal cord put together; indeed, these nerves are so substantial, powerful and significant that they are classified as a discrete nervous system – the Enteric Nervous System (ENS).

Scientists are only just beginning to appreciate the full potential of this nervous system. For example, it can operate on its own without requiring signals from the brain and its own "thoughts" can feed back and directly alter brain chemistry; but no one knows *exactly* how it does this.

And the food that we eat is just as complicated. Let's take as an example a common dish like beef stew and dumplings, one of my favourite winter suppers and a supremely nourishing Victorian culinary standard. Such a dish might have upwards of fifteen ingredients, with each of those ingredients consisting of thousands of molecules, many of which have neither been labelled scientifically, nor had their nutritional roles identified.[11] In the course of being cooked, eaten and metabolised, these molecules are combined, heated, chewed, broken down, absorbed and used within the body's cells. So in the end we're talking about the transformation, absorption and assimilation of many tens of thousands of molecule types. In other words, an astonishing number of chemical processes take place as a result of the preparation and consumption of even a relatively simple dish like beef stew and dumplings. To date, it has been virtually impossible to fully understand these chemical processes in scientific terms; they are far, far too extensive and complex.

Where dietary science *has* been very successful is in linking single nutrients to major diseases; i.e. where there is a deficiency of the nutrient, the disease arises. Examples of this include vitamin D and rickets, vitamin C and scurvy and vitamin B1 and beri beri. When the link between the nutrient and the disease was first identified, it seemed miraculous that such severe illness could be fixed with a simple dietary change.

The problem is that these dietary miracles have given us too much confidence in the overall insight of nutritional

---

11 Hounsome N *et al.* (2008) Plant metabolites and nutritional quality of vegetables. *Journal of Food Science* 73(4): 48-65.

science. In reality, when it comes to whole foods, groups of foods and their interactions with our very complex digestive systems and metabolisms, effective scientific understanding is distinctly lacking.

And that's where tradition comes in. For me, it has filled the gaps, enabling me to construct a truly comprehensive diet for health that is based on a small number of digestive concepts that are easily applied to climate, lifestyle, individual foods and food combinations. These concepts are symbiosis, secretion and motility – and I will use them both to describe digestive function and to analyse the best of food science.

- **Symbiosis** is all about the countless microbes that live in our guts help us to break down our food, and also produce vital nutrients.

- **Secretion** is the process by which the gut produces the chemical substances that break foods down so that they can be absorbed as they are moved along.

- **Motility** refers to the movement of the gut, when it is in harmony or when it is distressed.

These three digestive processes are interdependent and utterly influenced by the foods that we eat, the environments that we live in and the lifestyles that we lead. Together, they provide a comprehensive view of digestive function.

Symbiosis

As human beings, we are literally covered from top to toe, inside and out, with bacteria and other micro-organisms. Taking digestion as an example, it becomes clear that every human on the planet is his or her own little ecosystem. Our bodies are made up of around ten trillion cells but we have about ten times as many micro-organisms, or microbes, as they are sometimes called, in our guts; as much as two kilograms of the little fellows. These microbes can be bacteria, yeasts, fungi or larger animals (protozoa). They are known as the gut flora and may be good for health (symbiotic) or bad (pathogenic).

Naturally, in a healthy individual the vast majority of them are symbiotic (symbionts). Symbionts are absolutely vital to healthy living. Indeed, such is the role of these microbes in health that they have come to be known as the "forgotten organ". The crucial relationship that our bacteria have with health is one that is only just beginning to be appreciated scientifically. Recent DNA sequencing research concluded that human digestion is dependent on a *minimum* of 1000 species of bacteria, of which we probably have at least 200 in us at any one time.[12] What we don't know about our symbiotic bacteria is vast. What these bacteria look like and the potentially massive range of functions that they have within our bodies is beyond modern science. They are a vast, mysterious pool of little helpers.

Bacteria – our friends

So, what has been discovered in recent times about what

---

12 Qin J *et al.* (2010) A human gut microbial gene catalogue established by metagenomic sequencing. *Nature* 2010 Mar 4;464(7285): 59-65.

microbes do for our health? They clean our skin, help our babies to develop in the womb and line and protect our sinuses. And they form the bedrock of our digestion. Indeed symbiotic bacteria are so fundamental to health that a series of studies by Dr Martin Blaser, a New York microbiology professor, suggests that regular use of antibiotics that upset the balance of gut flora is linked to obesity as well as other major health problems such as allergies, inflammatory bowel disease and asthma.[13]

Those two kilos of symbionts in our guts are constantly working on our behalf to enhance our health by:

- helping us break down complex carbohydrates and sugars (fibres and the like)
- stimulating and supporting the immune system
- suppressing the development of harmful organisms
- producing useful nutrients like biotin and vitamin K that we aren't normally able to produce for ourselves
- helping to process fats
- developing the gut.

Bacteria – our enemies

We live in an age where there is, quite understandably, a fashion for cleanliness. After all, it is developments in hygiene and sanitation that have protected us from dreadful diseases such as polio, cholera, and infectious bacteria such as *Clostridium* and *Staphylococcus*, micro-organisms that have become infamous as hospital "superbugs". These diseases used to kill people by the million; now they are

13 Blaser M (2011). Antibiotic overuse: Stop the killing of beneficial bacteria. *Nature*, Aug 24;476(7361): 393-4. doi: 10.1038/476393a

much rarer in the Western world, largely because we have become cleaner.

This awareness of hygiene, combined with the awesome impact of antibiotics on infectious bacteria, has led to a philosophy of "anti-biosis" – humans constantly fighting pitched battles against other organisms – a philosophy that dominates medical thinking today. However, if we look back, for instance, to the case of the beta glucan-producing contaminant yeasts that so benefited the mid-Victorians, we may surmise that this philosophy of cleanliness has gone too far. Many, possibly most, micro-organisms are essential for health, a relationship known as "probiosis".

So, what are the implications of this for our diets? Despite the great unknowns around symbiotic interactions and digestion, there are some things that we do understand. It is inevitable that all these bacteria, including the good ones, are sourced from our environment and also from other humans in an important process called "seeding".

Seeding

Seeding takes place from conception. Some studies suggest that babies need bacteria for their growth and survival in the womb.[14] In other words, symbionts that are vital to health and development are working with us from the outset and they are picked up from the uterus. More bacteria are picked up at birth as the baby passes through its mother's vagina and into an area rich with digestive bacteria near her bottom. Further probiotic bacteria are then passed on through the breast milk.

The importance of this transmission of bacteria from

---

14 Wilks M (2007). Bacteria and early human development. *Early Human Development* 83, 165–170

mother to child and seeding of the baby's gut is revealed in statistics – babies born by caesarean section miss out on the vaginal bacteria and babies that aren't breast-fed miss out on bacteria from breast milk, leading to a higher incidence of disease in both groups. We are only just beginning to observe these vital relationships and much more research remains to be done in this area.

After birth and weaning, little children then continue to pick up symbionts from the floor and from the soil; even from pets. Again, the extent to which this seeding goes on to benefit us requires much study but, to take an example, it has been demonstrated that soil bacteria stimulate the release of extra serotonin, a key neurotransmitter, in the brain. Similarly, laboratory studies suggest that a range of major emotions, such as anxiety, are affected by the balance of our gut flora.[15] Muck actually makes us all happier![16]

So children instinctively seed their guts with little bacterial helpers, but what about us adults? Seeding is a process that we should continue throughout our lives. One way to achieve this is to grow our own food. Fruit and veg produced on an allotment, or even in a window box, in good organically managed soil, carry microbes that are beneficial to us – our exposure to this good, uncontaminated local dirt is great, and replicates the lives of the mid-Victorian market gardeners and children playing in the street.

We gain similar benefits from regularly consuming small

15 Bravo JA *et al.* (2011). Ingestion of Lactobacillus strain regulates emotional behavior and central GABA receptor expression in a mouse via the vagus nerve. *Proceedings of the National Academy of Science*, Sep 20;108(38): 16050-5. Epub Aug 29 2011.

16 Lowry CA, et al. (2007). Identification of an immune-responsive meso-limbocortical serotonergic system: Potential role in regulation of emotional behavior, *Neuroscience* doi: 10.1016/j.neuroscience.2007.01.067

amounts of live fermented foods such as sauerkraut, pickles and yoghurt, just like the mid-Victorians, who ate yoghurt and buttermilk, beer and pickled and preserved vegetables. Less attractive to the modern palate would be the pilchards that were "baulked" with salt in barrels and naturally preserved. Like herring, they were highly valued and a rich source of bacteria.

And whatever you think about pilchards, foods that are rich in bacteria are delicious and much cheaper than the sort of probiotic products that can be bought in the shops. Indeed, regular consumption of small amounts of fermented foods is one of the golden rules of healthy traditional diets, whether we're talking about the mid-Victorians, the Mediterraneans, the Chinese or the Japanese.

Time and time again, studies of the longest-living populations in the world reveal a fundamental place in their diets for these foods, such as the soy sauce, miso and fermented beans that the Chinese and Japanese rely on daily.

We should also not be too clean. Studies that compare the ultra-hygienic and disease-prone West Germans with the less scrubbed-up but healthier East Germans,[17] suggest that there is an optimum level of exposure to dirt. And it seems, with their access to soap, running water and toilets, the amount of dirt in the mid-Victorians' lives was about right for a balanced healthy lifestyle. To promote thriving internal communities of symbiotic bacteria, our modern diet should be considerably more earthy than it is now. We need to fundamentally change our diets and behaviour, and do away with obsessive scrubbing with highly toxic antibacterial agents.

---

17 Krämer U *et al.* (2010) Differences in allergy trends between East and West Germany and possible explanation. *Clinical & Experimental Allergy*, 2010 (40) 289–298.

In short, if we:

- ate more naturally preserved and fermented foods
- ate, played and worked more outside
- gathered more foods from hedgerows and wood-lands with their rich accompaniment of yeasts and bacteria
- just used normal soap rather than toxic industrial 'antibacterial' cleaners,

we would be an altogether healthier and happier bunch.

Artificial sweeteners

Recent research has shown the commonly used artificial sweetener sucralose to have significant destructive effect on gut symbionts.[18] The other major artificial sweetener aspartame is no better as once metabolised, it produces, among other chemicals, methanol, which is highly toxic to humans . Both products, which are used to sweeten "diet", "low-calorie", "sugar-free" and "weight loss" products, have been implicated in a wide range of debilitating diseases, including, interestingly, obesity.[19]

Stevia, a naturally occurring low-calorie sweetener – which has recently been declared "safe" for market, coincidentally at the same time as some major food companies came up with stevia-based products, has also had mixed

---

18 Mohamed B (2008). Splenda Alters Gut Microflora and Increases Intestinal P-Glycoprotein and Cytochrome P-450 in Male Rats. *Journal of Toxicology and Environmental Health*, Part A; 71 (21): 1415-29

19 For example, Nseir W *et al.* (2010). Soft drinks consumption and nonalcoholic fatty liver disease. *World Journal of Gastroenterology* Jun 7,16(21): 2579-88

reviews in terms of safety. My view is that stevia could damage health as it tricks the body's delicate hormonal systems into thinking there's a big sugar-based calorie hit in the offing when there isn't. The effect of this sweetener on symbionts is yet to be ascertained.

My advice would be to avoid all these sweeteners and stick to whole, natural foods instead.

Secretion

Food provides both the energy for and the substance of, our bodies. In order for it to fulfil these functions, it has to be first broken down into very small molecules in the gut, then absorbed through the membrane barrier that lines the stomach and intestines into the blood stream, and finally taken to where it is needed in the body.

To achieve the sort of molecule size that is easily absorbed into the blood stream, the typically large nutritional molecules of food have to be broken down many times over.

This is initially a mechanical process. Teeth chomp through the food and break it into little pieces. The breaking down then continues as a series of chemical processes involving enzymes, emulsifiers and other chemicals. It is worth talking about some of these as they will be referred to later in this book. They are also often misrepresented in fad diets!

Enzymes

Enzymes are proteins whose job it is to make chemical reactions happen more easily. Digestive enzymes are very specific for particular nutrient groups; there are enzymes that break down sugars and starches, enzymes that break down proteins, and so on. They do this by seeking out particular types of chemical bonds and snipping them to produce smaller and smaller molecules.

Enzymes are not only very specific in terms of the molecules on which they act, but also regarding the environment in which they work. For example, amylase, an enzyme that is secreted by the salivary gland, works best in the slightly alkaline warm conditions that are found in the mouth. Similarly, enzymes that are secreted in the stomach, where it is very acidic, work best in this acidity, and at body temperature.

Other chemical groups that aid breakdown in the gut include:

- the acid of the stomach itself
- emulsifiers which help to break insoluble chemicals into tiny droplets that enzymes can then act upon (bile is an example of a key emulsifier);
- alkalines – secreted in the bile, they are important as they neutralise the acid from the stomach. This protects the intestine and enhances the environment for the action of other secretions.

This range of digestive secretions breaks down the main nutritional macromolecules ("large molecules") that constitute the bulk of what we eat: carbohydrates, fat and protein. They are also instrumental in the release, modification and absorption of just about every other nutrient.

This has huge significance for the character of our diets because quite simply, *a dish is not balanced unless it stimulates secretion*. Indeed, as you will see when I discuss the digestion of fats shortly, if the ingredients of a dish are not tailored for its digestion then the results can be distinctly unpleasant. Just ask someone who suffers from IBS (Irritable Bowel Syndrome)!

The starting point for secretion stimulation comes before a meal has even begun, in the stimulation of appetite. Appetisers come in different forms. In Britain it might be a small glass of aromatic and sweet sherry or aromatic and bitter gin and tonic. In modern Germany herbal bitters are traditionally drunk before a meal, just as we drinkg angostura bitters in this country. In the Mediterranean salty olives or an intensely herbal fish or garlic soup are often eaten, and in China small salty fish or spicy shellfish or chicken wings (or feet!) are popular. All of these dishes and drinks stimulate secretion in preparation for the larger meal to come.

In the meal itself the key to managing secretion is the general *balance of flavours* in the dish. Spicy aromatics and bitterness are particularly good at stimulating secretion in the gut. Sourness is also important as it has a key role in the stimulation of bile secretion for the digestion of fats.

The disparity with the modern British diet could not be greater, packed as it is with salt and sugar, and with few other flavours. Contrast this with the mid-Victorian diet that was founded on bitter and aromatic herbs, and vegetable varieties that were considerably more bitter than modern ones. Spices, too, were enormously valued for their role in stimulating digestion.

The same beneficial factors are important in traditional Mediterranean and Asian cooking. Bitter herbs and spices such as basil, juniper, fenugreek and rosemary are used extensively in southern European cuisine and Chinese and Japanese cooking is characterised by the use of bitter greens. Similarly, it is no coincidence that the cornerstones of the

Chinese kitchen are aromatic spring onion and spicy ginger, garlic and chilli. They are there first and foremost for their stimulation of secretion and promotion of digestive strength. But these bitter, aromatic and spicy foods have another key function: they have expansive and moving qualities, which means that they stimulate motility.

Motility

In any natural context the essence of health is harmonious movement; as the ancients said "a stagnant stream becomes a putrid pond". The same principle applies to our digestion. If our blood keeps circulating and the food moves smoothly through our guts, then we are healthy. If blood and food stagnate, pain and disease will occur.

The need to achieve this slow, constant movement of food through our bodies is revealed in the structure of our guts. The digestive tract is essentially a long muscular tube, divided into separate parts with specific functions which are reflected in their form. Food is first chewed and passed down the oesophagus into the stomach, which is like a muscular bag. There, the food is stored and broken down, before slowly being pushed into the small intestine where it is further broken down and absorbed. It then passes to the colon and rectum, where water is reabsorbed and further digestive processes take place. Finally, waste products are expelled.

So we eat food, it is broken down, transformed, absorbed and finally excreted, a series of processes that rely on precisely controlled, smooth and constant movement from the top to the bottom of the gut. We need power for this movement, which is why the gut is so muscular.

Peristalsis

Gut muscles contract in sequential waves, pushing the food from one part of the digestive tract to the next, a precisely controlled process that is called peristalsis.

Peristalsis depends on the bewilderingly complex Enteric Nervous System (ENS). Like all complex systems, the ENS is easily disrupted and hence its function needs to be actively protected. If this function is not protected the result will be familiar in some form to most: trapped wind, bloating, abdominal and gastric pain, poor absorption. We can add the constipation and diarrhoea found in Irritable Bowel Syndrome (IBS) to the list of poor motility symptoms.

The pain from poor motility can be excruciating and crippling. And what's amazing about this process is that events in one part of the gut can cause loss of motility in another. For example, it is not unusual to experience bloating and trapped wind, largely in the colon (the "bottom end" of the gastrointestinal tract), having just eaten a meal. But this is a result of food that is still sitting in the stomach!

Most of us have experienced discomfort from poor motility; a significant proportion of the British population experiences these symptoms frequently. Our digestive systems are under constant daily strain as the three major factors that impact on motility are very commonplace. And since the functions of digestion are so intimately linked, the same factors often also impact on symbiosis and secretion. These three factors are *emotion, climate* and *diet.*

Emotion and digestion

Many of the nerves in the ENS are hitched up to gut muscles; they are "motor' nerves. These are the nerves that control peristalsis. So it is not surprising that the digestive tract is made up of very *nervous* organs. Indeed the stomach is second only to the heart and the brain in the secretion of a special group of molecules called neuropeptides, molecules that are central to *emotional* reactions. The result of this is that strong emotions such as stress and anxiety are able to inhibit motility.

The kind of constant, intense feelings associated with stress and anxiety activate the sympathetic nervous system, our so-called *fight, flight or freeze* nerves, which effectively shut down gut motility and secretion. Blood leaves the gut and surges to our arms and legs so that we can either defend our patch (fight), leg it (flight) or just plain panic (freeze). Warrior or coward, the result is not good for digestion, and I'm afraid to say that I spent many years in the panic category!

Mild examples of this sympathetic nervous reaction include pre-match butterflies and first-date appetite loss. But the constant nervous stimulation that we associate with stress can lead to extreme reactions like the nervous vomiting and severe gut cramps that affected me for years. In short, while stress and anxiety inhibit motility and secretion, *calm* protects them. It's not surprising then that in South-East Asian and Mediterranean societies eating times are reverentially cherished; and appropriate value given to the ritual of relaxation *and* nourishment. Indeed, even on long working days in China, a break is always taken at the right time of the day for a meal.

Contrasting lifestyles

Our working-class and middle-class Victorian forebears were calmer too. They took time to eat, read, talk and play games. They had much lower levels of stimulation and noise, no motorised traffic, no TV, smart phones, computer games or loud music. And they were much more spiritual than we are today, with a constant, reassuring belief in God and regular, community-building worship in the local church. There is strong evidence, including in the big Okinawa study, that community involvement and regular spiritual practice nurture calmness and self-confidence which in turn benefit digestion, health and longevity.

While the similarities between the Victorian lifestyle and values and those of healthy modern traditional societies, such as the Okinawans', are striking, the contrasts with modern Britain are stark. Many of us don't eat breakfast or lunch; or breakfast on the hoof, with working lunches and TV dinners increasingly the norm. This constant stress, stimulation and distraction erodes our digestive strength and motility, causing stagnation, fatigue and, in the long term, potentially life-threatening disorders such as cardio-vascular disease. As part of our healthy diet for Britain we definitely need to create *space* for eating and digestion, just like our ancestors did.

Case study

Nicky, 23, came to me with a constant stomach pain and the feeling that she had a lump in her throat. It was a nasty pain and could keep her awake at night. Nicky was also anxious and had suffered heavy periods for years. Initially doctors had found nothing wrong

---

and couldn't do anything, but then, before seeing me, she had consulted a nutritionist who put her on an "anti-candida diet". She was given a long list of foods to cut out, including red meat. From then her symptoms worsened and she became quite thin.

My diagnosis: poor blood supply to the heart and nervous system resulting in anxiety and restricted gut motility. I gave her herbs to strengthen and calm her and removed the restrictions on her diet. Now she could be calm around food, much better for motility. Rich foods like red meat were recommended(!) to nourish her blood and I emphasised the need for warm and cooked food and drink – again to protect motility.

Within two months Nicky was much happier, her pain had largely disappeared and she had gained 5kg to reach her healthy weight. This is a classic case where healing could only start with relaxation, but diet itself had to help her to relax. Only then could the gut move in a harmonious way.

Climate and digestion

Scientifically speaking, it's rather tenuous to relate climate with healthy digestion. But, in fact, throughout history humans have linked their digestive health to their surroundings. And the effects of climate on digestion are palpable today. Ever lost your appetite in heat and humidity, or felt tired after lunch on a cold, damp, drizzly day? Or woken up feeling stodgy with a poor appetite on a damp morning?

The Victorians may or may not have known about the advantages of their calmer lifestyles (although the likelihood is that they did, as the benefit of inner peace has been a perennial subject for health commentators, from Sun Si Miao to Hippocrates and Epicurus, all the way to Darwin). But they definitely knew about the impact of climate on health and digestion.

Connected to the elements

The Victorian connection with climate was much more intimate that it is in today's society. Their houses were draughtier and had no central heating. They didn't have the hard shell of a car to travel in, there was little heating and no air conditioning in the work place and schoolhouses were perishing in winter. In addition, clothes were much more expensive than they are now. For most people, hats weren't simply fashion, they were essential protection, as were boots, coats, scarves and neckerchiefs. Defensive action against wind, rain, damp, cold and the sun was vital health-enhancing behaviour.

Because of the ever-present awareness of the elements, rich, warming, cooked food was always prepared in spring, autumn and winter, and it was only on the warmer summer days that raw vegetables such as watercress might routinely be eaten – although the habit of regular salad eating was imported from warmer, drier France and largely practised by the aspiring and upper classes. The working class were much more likely to have lettuce in soup. Similarly cider was appreciated as a highly refreshing drink in the summer and around harvest time, but in the winter it was mulled with aromatic spices and served warm – a great soother and stimulant of motility! It is not just parochial eccentricity that has earned the British a reputation for warm beer: the practice is based on a sound health argument. Any Victorian who regularly drank cold beer would get frigid, stagnant guts and could fall ill.

These practices show us that the Victorians knew not only that they had to protect themselves from the external effects of climate, but that the effects of climate on digestion also had to be mitigated from within.

***

As we have seen, the gut's highly muscular nature means that it requires a prodigious blood flow to work effectively, hence digestion occupies up to 30% of our metabolism.

Unfortunately, however, the kind of cold and damp weather that is typical of Britain obstructs healthy circulation throughout the whole body, and since the gut requires such a high proportion of that circulation, its healthy and efficient function is compromised. This is why we lose our appetite in humid weather – the mugginess is literally blocking healthy movement of, and secretion within, the stomach. Similarly, the post-prandial tiredness that we often experience on cold, damp days is because extra resources have to be focused on digestion, leaving less blood and vitality for the rest of the body.

So it follows that the gut motility of a modern Briton is constantly being challenged. Ours is a wet, cool climate due to our northern latitude. Furthermore, many of us live in persistently damp locations such as drained marshes and moors, valley bottoms and basins, basement flats and houseboats. London, for example, was founded on estuarine marshland, and Bristol sits in the tidal Cumberland basin. Manchester is notorious for its constant rainfall, while parts of the mountainous Lake District rank as the wettest places in Britain. Even the drier east coast is cold and damp in global terms.

The impact of the climate on us is intense, yet our modern dietary culture and lifestyles are disconnected from it, in direct contrast to our ancestors of the nineteenth century, and other major dietary traditions. In China, for example, Sichuanese cuisine is famously spicy because of the persistent humidity of the region. The spice stimulates gut motility and causes sweating, which cools the body down. Further north the climate becomes colder and the food gets richer to compensate. It is always cooked and served hot to counter the predominant coldness while the flavours remain spicy to stimulate gut motility and compensate for the richness of the food.

Victorian cuisine was not renowned for its spice; on the contrary, it has something of a reputation for blandness. But this does it a disservice as it was highly aromatic and therefore strongly stimulated motility. The onion, leek and watercress that they ate so much of are all aromatic vegetables; and fresh aromatic herbs such as mint, coriander, rosemary and sage were a must in many staple dishes. Remember, also, that in those days vegetables had stronger flavours than our modern varieties do, as today they are cultivated for sweetness above all else. Spices were also valued and commonly used. Pungent black pepper was considered the "master spice". All of these ingredients could be grown at home or were readily available in the market. And, just as in northern China today, nearly all food was cooked and served hot.

To get back to a healthy diet, we need to re-establish our connection with climate, just like the mid-Victorians and the Chinese did. Cold salads and insipid clammy sandwiches should be made a thing of the past, and replaced with warm, nourishing, aromatic soups, stews and casseroles.

This theme of the importance of hearty, tasty, cooked and hot food is one that I will return to throughout the book. And, as you will see, many of my recipe commentaries relate the character of the dish, and the foods within it, to climate and season.

Bread, beer and dairy products

These three foods are worthy of note. While the Victorians consumed them in large quantities, they do not feature significantly in Chinese and Japanese diets. However, significantly, dairy and wheat products are far more commonly eaten in the north of China where the climate more closely matches our own – although there, unlike in modern Britain, they eat wheat and dairy products hot to compensate for the climate, and their dishes are typically heavily spiced to stimulate digestion. For the mid-Victorians it was the same: all food and drink was preferably consumed warm, and herbs and spices were widely used.

Furthermore, these foods were quite different in the mid-Victorian era, and often much healthier. Older, more digestible wheat varieties like spelt (see pp. 105, 201) were grown. Similarly milk, and all milk products, were unpasteurised and therefore more digestible.[20]

---

20 It is notable that a calf cannot thrive on pasteurised milk alone, it requires additional medication and supplements. The heat of pasteurisation fundamentally reduces the health properties of milk, and its digestibility, by killing symbiotic bacteria and structurally altering important proteins

Food choices to match emotion and climate

So far we have looked at the gut and how *emotion* and *climate* affect its functionality. Now we need to look at the way in which *specific foods* affect its workings, which foods are good, and which foods do us harm.

What we eat is, of course, what the digestive system exists to process, and the nature of the food to be processed can either help or inhibit the outcome. That is, the food can either break down easily to help the gut with its work, or it can be stubborn and sit in our bellies, like a lump.

Easily broken-down food enhances motility and takes the strain off secretion. The gut muscles don't have to work too hard, peristalsis is smooth and blood circulation is uninhibited: digestion is happy – everyone's getting along.

Overly rich, gloopy, sticky or over-fibrous food, and substances that quickly upset the balance of the gut and its symbionts – like the classic junk-food ingredients: refined sugar, artificial sweeteners and white wheat flour – have the opposite effect. These sorts of foods are either too hard to break down, or generate irritating chemicals, so that the gut has to work overtime to move them along. This causes a lot of strain. That's why many of us get a stomachache after Christmas lunch. Our digestion is overwhelmed, unlike in the gastric love-in that occurs after a healthy balanced meal. To deal with this, the body normally shuts down and goes to sleep, and gut motility suffers.

Of course, Christmas is a special day and should be celebrated as such. But if we eat in an unbalanced way all the time, the habit becomes a significant series of dietary errors. Even though the mid-Victorians ate huge amounts of food, most of it was selected from healthy food groups, and was then processed and combined in a way that was easily digested and beneficial to motility. This is why they did not experience the same gastric problems as we do today.

With respect to this, two groups of foods are particularly important, *fatty foods* and *raw fruit and veg*. Both of these food types are hard to digest as I will explain, yet both are essential ingredients for a healthy diet, making processing for digestibility absolutely vital to avoid diet-related illness.

Fatty foods

A balanced nutritious diet should include fatty foods, particularly the increasingly appreciated essential fatty acids (EFAs) that are abundant in foods like the herring that the mid-Victorians ate so much of. EFAs nourish the membranes of every cell in our bodies, they constitute the bulk of our nervous systems and they underpin important hormone manufacture and secretion. But fats are rich foods and they obstruct motility; they are really hard to shunt along the gut. Traditionally speaking, the answer to this problem has been to combine fats with flavours that help to break down the fat globules and molecules, and also to include flavours that stimulate motility to move the fat along the gut.

Sour is the flavour that helps to break up fats. Sour flavours tend to be acidic, such as the acetic acid in vinegar. They will raise the overall acidity of a dish and thus the acidity of the stomach, which stimulates the hormonal pathways that cause the release of bile into the small intestine. Bile has the effect of breaking up fat globules into smaller droplets, which can then be more easily moved, broken down and absorbed.

And sour, in turn, should be combined with the motility-stimulating flavours that help to move the fat droplets along the gut: spicy aromatics and bitterness. Indeed, these flavours *must* be combined with sourness in the digestion of fats, as sourness, though very good at helping to break down fats, is also astringent and so can have the effect of inhibiting motility.

Thus the expanding movement achieved by aromatics and spice and the downward movement achieved by bitterness work together to stimulate motility and balance out the inhibitory and contracting astringency of sourness.

This is why condiments that accompany fatty foods, such as the chutneys and pickles that the Victorians were fond of, are spicy and aromatic, sour and bitter. These flavours are essential companions to fatty foods as they stimulate the processes that break up fat and move it along the gut.

Compare this traditional approach to the way that we eat a modern-day high-street sausage roll or pie. Such products are normally eaten on their own, or sometimes with tomato ketchup that is so bland and sweet that it is more like jam. My mother's own traditional tomato ketchup recipe (p. 276) shows how ketchup should really taste: spicy, sour and not too sweet.

Fatty foods + sourness + spicy aromatics = good motility

- Sourness often comes from vinegar or lemon juice
- Aromatic spice and bitterness might come from juniper, allspice, turmeric, fenugreek, cumin, coriander, cayenne pepper and black peppercorns. (For example, the mint sauce that is traditionally served with fatty lamb is a simple combination of sour vinegar and aromatic mint.)

Raw foods and the importance of cooking

Raw foods present a different kind of digestive challenge to fatty foods. Human beings are not designed to digest raw food, and we never have been. As recent research by Professor Richard Wrangham and other prominent anthropologists demonstrates, humans and our hominid ancestors, have always cooked.[21] And this is reflected in the structure and function of our digestive systems.

So today we find raw food too tough; it sits around in our guts, challenging the balance of our symbionts, generating wind and obstructing motility. And, in the case of fruit and veg, much of it can pass through us undigested.

There are sound physiological reasons why humans find raw food hard to digest, which become obvious when we examine the digestive adaptations of other mammals.

Wild cats, for example, eat almost exclusively raw meat and bones, and their digestive systems are fit for purpose – extremely acidic in order to break down the fibrous connective tissue and kill the bugs that tend to fester in old meat. If our stomachs were that acidic, they would digest us from the inside out! And, like raw meat with its resilient connective tissue, raw fruit and veg have structures made up of molecules, cellulose and lignin, which are so tough that we simply cannot digest them.

Plant eaters in the animal kingdom get around this problem by relying very heavily on *fermentation*. All mammalian herbivores, for example, have regions of their anatomy that are enlarged for the storage of huge numbers of symbiotic bacteria. These bacteria then have a chance to

---

21 The anthropological detail of this theory is set out in *Catching Fire: How Cooking Made Us Human* by Richard Wrangham (2010). Profile Books

go to work on breaking down that tough, fibrous material, converting the plant matter into nutrients that the animals are then able to absorb and use.

For cows this fermentation vat is the stomach, giving them their characteristic barrel bellies. For rabbits and horses it's the caecum, the so-called hind gut, which contains a mixture of friendly fermenters. Indeed, rabbits even eat their own stools so that they get a chance to ferment their food twice.

Closer to us on the evolutionary tree, primates have long intestines to house bacteria and to aid absorption: this is why they sport pot bellies. In addition, like herbivores that chew the cud, primates spend a long time chewing to break down the physical structures of the food.

All of these behavioural and anatomical adaptations mean that different species tend to be very specialised in what they eat, as they are built to digest a relatively narrow range of foodstuffs.

Humans, by contrast, have a hugely varied diet, if we consider what is eaten in different parts of the globe. Roots, seeds, fruits, vegetables, worms, grubs, insects, seafood, birds and a wide range of mammals are all included. No animal on the planet matches humans in terms of the variety of foods that they consume. And yet, bizarrely, if we ate large amounts of any of this food raw we would get a mighty stomachache or even food poisoning.

To avoid this kind of digestive stress we have a key biological adaptation – we transform our food by peeling, chopping, cooking and external fermentation.

The use of these processes means that effectively humans have always eaten their food *pre-digested*; we have to because, in digestive terms, we are weaklings. We simply can't cope with tough, fibrous food. The studies by Professor

Wrangham and others explain why this should be.

Since our stomachs aren't that acidic, our guts aren't that long and we don't have a specifically enlarged "fermentation vessel" part like other mammal plant eaters, we can't seem to handle the food that other mammals eat, in its raw state. However, our energy-hungry brains, which require a quarter of all our energy, place an intense burden on our relatively weak digestions. No other animal thinks so much.

Therefore, cooking our food has always underpinned our survival as human beings. Cooking means that we can eat food faster without having to chew as much, since the heat of cooking breaks up larger molecules and structures in the food. We can also get more energy from it when it gets into our guts because we are relieved of the need to spend energy on breaking down remaining complex chemical structures. This is a great benefit as digestion already consumes a third of our metabolic energy.

If we ate only raw food, our guts would consume even more energy digesting *and* we'd have to chew for at least *six hours a day*. What is so fascinating about this is that *Homo sapiens* is not the only species that ever cooked. Our ancestors, the hominids, did too. In other words, we evolved cooking: it's all that we've ever done.

Appreciation of these biological facts is very important because, while healthy motility and symbiotic balance underpins the digestion of all mammals alike, each species achieves these balances in a different way, through different behaviours, different gut structures and different food choices. To be healthy, we need to make uniquely human choices: that means cooking our food.

In modern Britain there is a view, fuelled by fad diets, that substantial consumption of raw fruit and vegetables is healthy. This view is simply wrong and nearly completely at odds with the mid-Victorian diet and the traditional diets of the world's healthiest people today. As has already been discussed, the mid-Victorian working-class diet was mostly cooked, not just because the climate was cold and hot food was therefore more attractive, but also because cooked food is more digestible and thus kinder to motility and absorption. Fuel was expensive – these hard-working people would not have cooked if they didn't have to!

Similarly, traditional Chinese and Japanese diets are nearly all cooked, regardless of the prevailing climate, and in cases where raw food, such as sushi, is served, there are always strong spicy accompaniments, such as wasabi and pickled ginger to stimulate motility; just as we British traditionally combine ham with mustard or rare beef with horseradish.

It is true that more raw food is eaten as part of the Mediterranean diet, but this is largely a matter of climate. The Mediterranean climate is predominantly hot and dry, presenting much less of a challenge to motility than our cold and damp weather. And Mediterraneans still eat almost exclusively cooked food in winter when the weather is colder and wetter – after all, they're human too, so the principles are the same...

So, if the scientific and anthropological evidence clearly indicates that we should not be eating a diet mainly composed of raw food, why do so many restaurant menus, health retreats and books still advocate its consumption?

Raw foodism is a classic example of a fad that is based on scientific *language*, but not on sound scientific arguments. To clarify, here are the key claims of the "raw food" diet and explanations as to why they are inaccurate:

CLAIM: Raw food preserves vital enzymes, otherwise denatured by cooking

Raw foodism suggests that humans need the help of enzymes in food to be able to digest it effectively. There is no good scientific evidence for this claim. Enzymes are proteins that are mostly denatured by our own stomach acid. The food-derived enzymes are in fact digested by the special protease enzymes secreted in our stomachs (which are not denatured by the stomach acid as they are specifically adapted to working in a very acidic environment). Rather than the enzymes helping us to digest, we digest the food enzymes themselves! Any "vital enzymes" which survive the stomach to get to the small intestine, and which aren't locked up in indigestible raw food material, probably would not work properly there either, as the small intestine is an intensely alkaline environment which would also distort and denature the plant enzymes. It is also quite possible that as our body temperature (around 37°C), is higher than the ambient temperature to which most plants that we eat are adapted, the plant enzyme function would be compromised. So any help that we might get from "vital enzymes" would be minuscule to the point of insignificance relative to the massive amount of digestive enzymes that we already produce for ourselves.

CLAIM: Raw food is more nutritious as cooking destroys nutrients

Cooking does destroy nutrients, but it also makes them more available than they would be from raw food, by breaking down the tough or fibrous structures of the food and allowing for easier absorption. So in real terms, cooked food is more nutritious than raw food. A specific example of a nutrient that is less easily absorbed from raw food because of its indigestibility is carotene from carrots.

In addition, cooking helps to enhance the nutrient content of foods by forming new essential nutrients, such as lycopene from tomatoes.[22]

CLAIM: Raw food benefits health through detoxification of the body

Although it sounds like it, "detoxification" is not a scientific term. I believe that detoxification is a term that is used to explain away the fact that people feel awful on a raw-food diet because it is not healthy and sustaining. If worried about specific toxicity, why not eat food that is fresh,

---

22 For example: Pellegrini N *et al* (2009). Effect of domestic cooking methods on the total antioxidant capacity of vegetables. *International Journal of Food Sciences and Nutrition*, Vol. 60 (s2): 12-22. Hornero-Mendez D & Minguez-Mosquera M (2007). Bioaccessibility of carotenes from carrots: Effect of cooking and addition of oil *Innovative Food Science & Emerging Technologies* 8 (3): 407-412

from non-toxic agriculture and cooked by boiling or steaming so that no toxins develop in the first place? Ironically, raw-food diets may actually be more toxic than cooked diets. Cooking destroys toxins: this is why we cook potatoes and beans. Also raw food upsets the symbiotic balance, which is why it makes us fart so much; and when the gut flora struggles it produces irritant chemicals that have a toxic effect.

So, in what instance could people feel healthier on a raw-food diet? I believe the most common explanation for a person feeling better on a raw-food diet is that when they embark on it they are also giving up booze and junk food. The Western Diet is so bad that most people will feel better when they adopt a relatively fresher and more wholesome alternative. But the perceived benefits do not last. The Giessen Raw Food study conducted in Germany (which has a northern temperate climate like ours), showed a high proportion of raw-foodists suffering low body mass and chronic fatigue. Fifty per cent of the women on the diet ceased to menstruate and men suffered low libido; there was a very high level of infertility among both men and women.[23] None of these are indicators of good health.

The raw-food movement started in the desert states of the southern USA as a Caucasian adaptation to the searing and desiccating climate. Raw vegetables were felt to have a hydrating and cooling effect and were considered a significant

---

23 These statistics, together with extensive explanations repudiating the raw foodists' arguments, are detailed at length in *Catching Fire: How Cooking Made Us Human* by Richard Wrangham the Harvard anthropologist credited with highlighting the importance of cooking to humans

remedial foodstuff. But the same principle should not be adopted in Britain; this dietary zeitgeist is not appropriate for our cold and damp temperate climate at all.

4.

The Flavour Principle

I introduced the theory of the properties of flavours above, in my discussion of digestive function and the promotion of healthy symbiosis, secretion and motility. The basic flavours, just as a reminder, are as follows:

- natural sweetness to nourish symbionts
- sourness to cut through fats
- bitterness, spice and aromatics to stimulate secretion and motility
- salt to stimulate appetite.

I will now explain why they play such a vital role, and how we can best make use of them. In the days before the development of nutritional chemistry, flavour was the main tool for the analysis and classification of foods. Individual foods or combinations of foods were said to strengthen, invigorate, cleanse, refresh, decongest, calm, move, heat, cool, cause sweating and nourish the body, all according to their flavour or blends of flavours. This was the traditional language of diet and one that was common to medieval Britain, Victorian Britain, Ayurveda (the traditional health practice of India), ancient and modern China and beyond.

In today's Britain we have nearly entirely lost touch with

the health properties of flavours. Yet they are just as relevant as analytical tools in the bewilderingly complex chemistry of foods, digestion and metabolic processes as they always were.

It would be impossible to summarise in a properly scientific way the interaction of all the chemicals in the foods that we ingest, or how they react with us once we've eaten them. There are simply too many chemicals and processes to take into account, in any practical or accessible way. What we can do, however, is continue to base our dietary system on flavour, as humans have done for millennia.

And, actually, flavour analysis *is* scientific in its way, since it is not exclusively traditional/anecdotal. All the nutritional chemical classes have their own distinctive flavours (acids are sour, alkaloids are bitter, aromatic oils are aromatic, sugars are sweet, glutamates are savoury) and flavours do reflect the chemical constituents of food, and hence their actions in terms of health, accurately.

There are slight variations in the classification of flavours in different countries and traditions but the system I have found easiest to relate to is the Chinese tradition of five flavours:

- sweet
- salty/savoury
- sour
- bitter
- spicy/aromatic.

There is a good reason for this: the Chinese literature describing these flavours and the foods that possess them is extensive, very detailed and continues to be written and updated to this day; in contrast to our own British literature and traditions which have been buried since the Enlightenment movement of the eighteenth century and seem to be only of academic interest today. For the purposes of a British diet, the Chinese five-flavour system is close enough to pre-Enlightenment British flavour analysis, which was itself based on ancient Greek literature and philosophies.

What those forebears had was a deep familiarity with flavours and the foods that possessed them. This familiarity was then applied to food production, procurement, combination, cooking and consumption, with great effect in terms of creating a healthy diet. What we have to do now as part of a healthy diet is develop the same degree of knowledge through examining each flavour category in much greater detail.

Flavour – science and tradition

For a long time scientists have recognised four flavour categories: bitter, salty, sour and sweet. Chinese tradition adds spicy/aromatic to this and Ayurveda (the traditional health practice of India) a further category – astringent.

Ancient Greek and Roman medical commentators, including Hippocrates and Galen (Galen was a Greek living in Rome), on whose work the institutional Western European dietetic traditions were largely based, recognised as many as nine flavours but their categories still displayed similar characteristics to those of the Chinese.

Another flavour, *umami*, was officially recognised in 1908. This is the taste of glutamates and nucleotides, but, since umami is basically a flavour enhancer that acts on salt in particular, it tends not to occupy its own category in traditional systems. However, to take account of the importance of savoury flavours such as umami in cooking, not just for salt, I refer to the salty category as salty/savoury in this book.

Interestingly, receptors on the tongue for another taste that is not included in traditional systems have just been discovered: *fat*. This emphasises the importance of this nutrient in human evolution and health. Again, I will not discuss fat as a distinct flavour category as it is relatively bland and, like umami, would either act as a flavour enhancer in general or be classified as savoury (or sometimes sweet, especially when cooked).

Sweet

We all have an instinctive love for this flavour, which exists for good reason. Sweetness reflects the sugar content of foods, which provides the calories to sustain us in our day-to-day lives. This ongoing energetic sustenance means that in traditional terms sweetness is known as the *strengthening* flavour – the one that more than any other builds strength, and digestive strength in particular. As such, it is ideal for staple foods – those that form the foundation and bulk of your healthy diet. If you look at the table of staple foods (page 106), you will see that they are usually slightly sweet in nature. They might be referred to as sweet and "bland". In other words, they are sweet, without being too sweet.

This balance of sweetness with blandness is particularly important for our symbiotic bacteria which we carry with us are like a special culture that needs nurturing and main-taining. Symbiotic bacteria require a certain amount of complex sugars, at a certain rate, to flourish. The benefit of good sweet-bland staples is that they provide that perfect amount and type of complex sugars that our symbiotic bacteria need. If they don't get enough of these foods, our symbionts die off and we become weak.

The balance is delicate, however. If we eat too much very sweet-tasting *refined* sugar, then disease-causing (patho-genic) micro-organisms such as candida yeasts grow at a dangerous rate, edging out our symbiotic bacteria, weak-ening our digestion and making us ill; not to mention the havoc that such sugar also plays with our vital hormonal balances, particularly those of insulin, resulting in today's extraordinary national levels of obesity and diabetes. The ubiquity of refined sugar, fructose syrups and the like means that the sweet flavour is the most abused in modern Britain, a practice that began over a century ago with the nutritional decay of the late Victorians.

In the 1870s, refined sugar became cheap and widely available, as did white wheat flour, which quickly turns to sugar as we eat it. These two disease-causing foods rapidly became staples in the British diet, causing a precipitous decline in the nation's health.

Today virtually all industrially processed food is crammed with sugar, because food manufacturers know that sweet-ness creates compulsion. The attraction to sweetness that is part of our hard-wiring has made us like moths flying to a candle. In many cases, the knowledge that we can constantly eat sweet food literally dominates our senses. It did for the late Victorians and, in the form of today's Western Diet, it's hammering us too.

Despite this sorry tale, handled with care, the sweet flavour can be used to enhance health. Sweetness is the flavour of staple products such as oats, rye, barley, older wheat varieties (such as spelt) and potatoes, and so underpins a healthy diet. And as it is the strengthening flavour, it is particularly important for recuperation and convalescence. Chicken soup has come to be known as "Jewish penicillin" for good reason; the light sweetness of a chicken broth, made with barley and a few root vegetables, makes it the ideal tonic food for the immune system as it battles infection, not to mention the boost it gives our symbionts, which help us in the task.

More than any other flavour, sweetness can sustain, recover and create health. But use it wisely, for it can also destroy health. It is up to us to manage this balance.

Sweet summary

- Stimulates and strengthens digestion
- Fuels metabolism
- Nourishes symbiotic bacteria

N.B. Food should only be slightly sweet; refined sugar and artificial sweeteners are very destructive

---

Case study

Sinead, 28, came to me feeling "out of balance". She had a history of anxiety and depression and had previously taken antidepressant medication over an eight-year period. She was also suffering from thrush following a dose of antibiotics.

To improve her mood it was necessary to reduce the stagnation in her gut and to strengthen her – as a mentor once said to me, "95% of depression is a form of tiredness". I got her to eat a richer diet with plenty of healthy protein and fat so that her brain and heart had constant nourishment. She cooked with more mild aromatic herbs and spices to stimulate motility. I also gave her tonic and moving herbs to amplify these effects.

To treat the thrush it was necessary to strengthen her digestive symbionts, to keep her body flora in balance. I got her to cut out refined sugars and foods that are naturally rich in sugars (such as malt), and to greatly reduce her intake of wheat. The thrush disappeared but we discovered over time that it would return with even the tiniest intake of sugar.

Her mood also improved and stabilised and today she feels perky, much to everyone's enjoyment as she is a wonderfully fun and lively character!

Salty/savoury

This flavour is dominated by one chemical: salt, an ingredient that rightly gets a bad press these days. There is too much of it in the Western Diet, as it is added in prodigious quantities to just about every food product available.

Why? Because, just like the sweetness of refined sugar, we crave it. Unfortunately, high salt consumption is linked to raised levels of heart disease, high blood pressure, dementia and strokes, and this is why there are so many warnings against eating lots of salty food.

But this has not always been the case. Traditionally speaking, salt is said to play a role in health. We talk about people "earning their salt"; there was a time when it was a rare and treasured flavour enhancer and medicinal substance. Certain foods, like seeds, were – and still are – processed with salt in order to stimulate the urinary system and strengthen digestion and the constitution.

For example black sesame seeds are widely used in Japanese and Chinese cooking as a traditional tonic, and women who feel weak and unable to regulate their body temperature after birth are given salt-fried black sesame seeds to fortify them.

Similarly, salt-fried aromatic seeds are used to stimulate digestive function in Ayurvedic medicine.

So how should we approach salt in terms of our diet? Generally speaking, we should seek to limit it to a small but satisfying quantity; commercially produced bread, breakfast cereals, snacks and ready meals are all loaded with it and our palates have come to expect large amounts of salt in our food. Shockingly, many foods for babies and children also have added salt. In modern Britain we don't have to seek out salt… salt will find us!

However, if you get into the habit of eating freshly prepared and cooked food, you will find that you need to add only a little salt for taste. It will then act solely as a flavour enhancer and not as an addictive agent. Indeed, probably the best approach is to do as the mid-Victorians did: instead of adding salt to food as it is cooked, have a little pile of it on the edge of the plate to dip into as and when it is necessary.

It is also worth noting that some types of salt are better than others – a traditionally produced sea salt gives much more flavour and nutrition, and therefore smaller quantities are required than of the cheap mass produced stuff.

The use of naturally salty/savoury foods is discussed later in the book. Generally speaking they fall into three categories, all of which tend to be rich in mineral salts and/ or umami: foods from the sea, deeply savoury foods and flavour-enhancing sauces and condiments. Here are some examples:

From the sea	Deeply savoury foods	Flavour enhancers
Anchovies	Celery stalk	Brown sauce
Mussels	Duck	Mushroom ketchup
Oysters	Pigeon	Soy sauce
Seaweed	Pork	Worcester sauce

Salty summary

- Can nourish the constitution *in small quantities*
- Enhances other flavours
- Stimulates appetite
- Moves the bowel

N.B. Use a small amount of really good quality salt and watch out for added salt in pre-prepared foods.

Sour

In comparison with sweet and salty/savoury, there is relatively little sour in our diets.

Traditionally speaking, sour is the *cooling* and *refreshing* flavour, an ideal antidote to our overheated constitutions and lifestyles in the West. Hence, sourness in the diet is said to be *calming* and can be advantageously used in times of stress. Sometimes we talk about being "liverish", that is, feeling obstructed both digestively and emotionally. The dietary answer is to eat more sour foods, which stimulate the liver and gall bladder.

Some classic British examples of sour foods used to this end are crab apple, damson, hawthorn, sloe and rose hip. Historically, these grew in profusion in hedgerows and were prepared as sauces, jellies, purées or syrups to soothe and move the gut and liver. Sourced from nearby European countries and with a long history in British cuisine, citrus fruits such as lemon and lime have a similar role.

Further afield there are many such approaches to the sour flavour. An example of this is the sour or Chinese plum, *ume* in Japanese. Just as we once did with our damsons and sloes, this wonderful fruit is variously juiced, pickled, preserved, smoked and made into wine. The juice is light, sour and refreshing, especially when consumed in summer to counter the affect of heat on the body. The pickles and preserves have a more intense sourness and this makes them particularly useful when consumed after meals, especially heavy fatty meals, to disperse the fats and to aid digestion.

Similarly, in China, hawthorn is combined with cinnamon and other digestive herbs and made into sour sweets to be eaten after meals. These are widely available and particularly popular with children.

In Britain, because of our cold climate, it is essential that we eat a decent amount of rich food. Rich, fatty food provides the calories that we need to get through long winter days while also enhancing satiety so that we avoid the hunger cravings that so commonly affect those who struggle with their weight. In the age of the calorie-controlled diet the idea that rich food actually helps us reduce our body weight might seem counter-intuitive; but study after study confirms this phenomenon. Those who eat a rich meal like scrambled eggs for breakfast have lower, more stable body weights. As I explain in greater detail in Chapter 8, the reason for this is simple: rich food fills you up. So, if you eat it, you'll want to eat *less overall*.[24]

However, as we have already discussed, because of its high fat content, rich food is harder to digest. This is the reason why eggs are often associated with digestive intolerance: the high fat content of the yolk obstructs gut motility. Yet, consumption of eggs should not inevitably lead to a stomachache, as our scrambled egg recipe (p. 230) demonstrates; by combining the eggs with sour tomatoes to help break up the fats, and aromatic spices to stimulate motility, the digestive system gets the help that it needs.

This example reminds us that, as part of an easily digestible British diet, we should always accompany rich meals with sour ingredients, condiments and dressings, just like they used to in mid-Victorian times.

Here are some classic combinations that follow the principle of combining the sour flavour with rich and fatty foods:

---

24 Ander Wal J *et al* (2008). Egg breakfast enhances weight loss. *International Journal of Obesity* 32, 1545–51

- Cheese and pickle
- Coconut milk and lime
- Duck and orange
- Lamb and mint sauce (made with vinegar)
- Pie and chutney – chutney fruits include apple, apricot, grape, kiwi, mango and plum
- Olive oil and lemon or balsamic vinegar
- Pork and apple or cider
- Salmon and sorrel.

Sour summary

- Stimulates bile release to break down rich foods
- Calms
- Use in winter to cut through the richer diet
- Use in summer to refresh when hot

Bitter

Bitterness is the most neglected of the five flavours; unsurprising considering the bad press that this particular flavour has had over the years. And such negativity seems to be widespread. In Britain "bitterness" is associated in emotional terms with resentment, dissatisfaction, even anger; while the Chinese, despite the breathtaking variety and prevalence of bitter foods and herbal preparations in their diets, still talk about *chi ku*, literally "eating bitterness", to describe hardship.

And yet, the bitter flavour was once much loved in Britain, and still is in other parts of the world. Bitter greens such as dandelion, chicory, lettuce, kale and chard were cherished by the mid-Victorians, but are largely neglected by us today.

Historically, the varieties of bitter vegetable that were grown in Europe, from cucumber to cabbage, were more diverse and much more bitter than they are today – the bitterness has been bred out of them in favour of sweetness.

This change is to our detriment as bitterness is a profoundly *medicinal* flavour – indeed, bitter is arguably the *most* medicinal flavour, a key ingredient in a wide range of phytochemicals with antibacterial, antiviral, anti-inflammatory and diuretic properties. Therefore, nearly every traditional herbal remedy tasted, and tastes, bitter. That's why Mary Poppins sang "a spoonful of sugar helps the medicine go down", and why medicine has always been a "bitter pill to swallow"!

The bitterness of many medicinal foods is something that is appreciated in Asia to this day. As an example, let's consider the bitter melon or *goya*, a vegetable that is hugely popular in ultra-healthy Okinawa. Its medical properties are said to be founded on its bitterness. Bitter melon is widely consumed in Pakistan, India, China and Japan to cool the body down and balance the heating effects of climate and a strongly spiced diet. It has great remedial properties: it regulates the bowel, a result of its bitter constituents stimulating excretion and motility, and it also moistens and protects the lungs.

Incidentally, when the Chinese talk figuratively about *chi ku* – eating bitterness – this is not a reference to the bitter flavour *per se*, but to forced overconsumption of this powerful flavour; even with today's runaway global sugar consumption, bitter foods are still much loved in Asia!

The cooling property of bitterness has led the Chinese to say that "bitter drains heat from the heart". Thus bitterness is said to have a *calming* effect, especially when the weather is hot. Traditionally, this has encouraged a habit of consuming more bitter food in the height of summer. It is said to enhance sleep, reduce irritability and help to prevent the onset of "liverishness". Like the sour flavour, the use of this cooling property also benefits us in the West as our hectic and stressed lifestyles get us "hot under the collar"!

In damper weather, bitters are said to compensate by *drying out* the body, as well as stimulating movement of the bowel to counter damp's stagnating effect. This makes bitterness particularly suited to the British weather.

So bitter is actually an incredibly versatile flavour. And the British should be proclaiming its nutritional power from the rooftops, rather than consigning it to the odd leafy green, condiment or aperitif as we currently do.

The nutritional celebration of bitterness is not as hard as it may sound: bitterness can be found in many foods. Leafy greens tend to be bitter and grow all year round in one form or another. Similarly, seasonal greens, courgette, cucumber, aubergine and broccoli are all classified as bitter vegetables.

The most significant bitter substance of all, however, is not a food but a drink – tea. Tea, an infusion of the leaves of the *Camellia sinensis* plant, is consumed in huge quantities by people worldwide, including, of course, the British. And its health properties are extensive,[25] which means that, combined with its ubiquity, it is arguably the world's greatest medicine.

25 See *Green Gold The Empire Of Tea* by Alan and Iris Macfarlane and Dr John Briffa's *Escape the Diet Trap* p202

Tea

With regards to digestion, tea is hugely significant and versatile. It regulates digestion as its astringent tannic acid protects against diarrhoea, while its bitter components (such as alkaloids) stimulate the bowel to counter constipation. Meanwhile, antibacterial agents maintain the balance of our symbionts and protect our teeth from bacteriogenic erosion. No wonder then that tea has been the traditional mealtime beverage in China for countless generations and was the favourite domestic tipple of the mid-Victorians.

Tea has a pivotal role our lives, dictating the rhythm of our days, getting us going in the morning and lubricating our breaks and mealtimes.

However, all is not rosy in the British tea garden. As is the case with so many foods in modern times, we have found a way of largely negating its health benefits, through the addition of two miscreants, milk and our old enemy sugar.

Neither of these ingredients is added to tea in China, rather it is drunk pure, in green or black forms (although the Chinese call black tea *hong cha* which translates as "red tea"). Our British preference is for tea "white" (through the addition of milk) and sweet.

Sugar, of course, rots our teeth and disturbs symbiotic balance so its impact is obviously and directly opposed to the natural digestion-enhancing effects of tea. Milk is similar. Its proteins bind out the astringent and bitter tannins, and neuter other chemicals too, such as the catechins that protect our hearts. This means that compared with pure teas, our typical British cuppa is a rather insipid brew.

There are ancient tea-drinking cultures that routinely drink milky tea (what the Chinese call *nai cha*), most notably the Tibetans, who add milk and butter to their infusions. But there is a good reason for this. The Tibetan climate is so cold that they have to consume a rich diet day in day out to stay warm, and for religious reasons they eat little or no meat, hence the addition of butter in the tea. Furthermore, as the Tibetan plateau is so dry that digestion is relatively unobstructed, they can get away with consuming the rich drink without excessive digestive impact. In other words, combining the rich dairy products with digestion-enhancing tea is a necessity for the Tibetans. For us, with our damp climate, this is a liberty that we shouldn't take. Persistent dampness means that we need the tea's dark bitterness much more than we need the milk that we add to it!

Tea provides a cautionary tale for us all. There is a view that sugary white tea powered the industrial revolution, as a calorie-starved proletariat added protein and carbohydrate to their favourite pick-me-up. But this was simply not the case. The increasing availability of food into the mid-nineteenth century meant that most people had plenty to eat, and their tea-drinking habit from this point was driven more by culture and compulsion than necessity. Rather, as cheap sugar flowed in from the Caribbean colonies, tea got sweeter and sweeter, in step with the demise of the late Victorians.

Some say that Queen Victoria enjoyed the symbolism of sweet white tea, uniting as it did the three corners of Empire, sugar from the Caribbean, tea from the Raj and milk from Britain. But, as her reign progressed, her humble subjects' teeth fell out, meaning that they could literally no longer chew the huge quantities of fruit and vegetables that had sustained Britain only one generation before.

Perhaps this is one area where sentimentality might do us more harm than good. I don't expect for one moment to change Britain's tea-drinking culture in the round. We are so deeply attached to it. But ignorance isn't bliss, and I have come to greatly love the immense variety and aromas of green teas, white teas (leaves picked when they are still very young and white in appearance), fermented teas (red, brown and black), and their health-enhancing properties.[26]

If we were to change one thing it should be to stop putting sugar in our tea. Adding milk isn't great, but I don't want to labour this point; its effects on health are far less harmful than adding sugar.

---

26 On a subtle level different types of tea impact on digestion in different ways. Too much black tea, especially from tea bags, can weaken digestion – it is very astringent so in excess it inhibits motility, while its strong tannins can affect symbionts. Green tea is lighter and more aromatic, so more digestion friendly in large quantities. More aromatic still is jasmine tea; the oils from the jasmine flowers stimulate motility

Here is a list of everyday bitter foods to include in your diet, the majority of which were relished by our mid-Victorian ancestors:

Artichoke	Basil
Broccoli	Bay leaf
Buckwheat	Chervil
Celery	Chives
Chard	Coffee
Chicory	Dill
Dandelion	Fenugreek seed
Dark chocolate/cocoa	Juniper berry
Kale	Lemon zest
Lettuce	Marjoram
Millet	Mustard
Parsnip	Oregano
Rocket	Parsley
Rye	Rosemary
Watercress	Tea

Bitterness summary

- Moves the gut and stimulates secretion and motility
- Helps push food down the bowel
- Counters the pathogenic effects of dampness
- Cools and calms

Spicy/aromatic

The British are famous for their love of spicy and aromatic foods and curry in particular, a culinary relationship that was established long ago.

The use of ginger, cinnamon, nutmeg, cloves, galangal, cubebs, coriander, cumin, cardamom and aniseed is well documented among the upper classes during the reign of Richard I (1157–1199), and it was under the instruction of Richard II (1367–1400) that the famous cookbook *The Forme of Cury* was written. By Elizabethan times, curry had become even more widely appreciated: Gervase Markham's *The English Housewife* contained a recipe similar to a dish served in the court of Emperor Jahangir in India.

With the expansion of the empire in Victorian times, and ready availability of exotic ingredients, such as turmeric, cumin and coriander, people of all classes began to consume more spicy and aromatic foods, which, as they already knew, had significant health benefits. Indeed, the use of these spices actually helped to save money as the they routinely curried meat to extend the shelf life of leftovers.

Move the clock forward and you will see that even in modern times, spices and aromatics are not necessarily underrepresented in our diets. Some of us eat loads of them. The problem is that we don't eat them fresh enough, we don't combine them with the right foods, such as fatty foods that challenge motility, and we don't use them sufficiently to mitigate the effects of our climate. For, in our cool, damp climate, spicy flavours and aromatic oils are vital.

These are the *moving* flavours, and many spicy and aromatic foods have a *warming* quality, and are therefore ideal for stimulating gut motility, which is slowed by our cold and wet weather. When digestion stagnates, causing symptoms like trapped wind and poor appetite, dietary traditions throughout the world use spicy and aromatic foods like fennel seeds as a matter of course to get it moving again –and so did the British up to a few decades ago; now, however, we seem to rely on proton-Pump inhibitors, antacids and laxatives.

Not all of the spicy and aromatic foods warm, however; coriander, marjoram and mint leaves actually have cooling and refreshing properties. This makes them ideal for balancing out warming foods like lamb and chilli, and is why the classic British combination of lamb with mint sauce works, and why the Thais use so much fresh coriander leaf in their curry broths.

Spicy and aromatic foods have another huge health benefit for the British. It is well documented that the stagnant, damp air that many of us have to endure damages the health of the lungs, especially when it is combined with pollution. Spicy and aromatic foods are the principal dietary method of combating this effect. The oils in these foods help the lungs to move, to expand and contract freely, and to shift phlegm. This is why traditional cough linctus and decongestants are intensely aromatic.

Considering the astonishing incidence of lung disease in this country (around four people a day die from asthma in the UK), spicy and aromatic foods are vital in our diets.

Aromatic and spicy foods have a range of intensities. The chilli and pepper that characterise strong curries and some Sichuanese dishes are at the top end of the scale and are too strong for our purposes. In the long term, regular consumption of large amounts of food this spicy damages health as it irritates membranes and causes inflammation. In fact, during my time in a Sichuanese hospital I was shown a distinct category of patient who had overdone it on the famously spicy diet. Not to be copied!

Instead, we need to include *mild* aromatic foods, herbs and spices as staples in our diet. Here are some common examples:

Vegetables	Spices	Leafy Herbs
Celeriac	Cardamom	Basil
Fennel bulb	Cinnamon	Celery
Garlic	Coriander seed	Coriander leaf
Leek	Cumin	Mint
Onion	Fennel seed	Oregano
Radish	Mustard seed	Rosemary
Watercress	Paprika	Thyme

Spicy/aromatic summary

- Stimulates motility and circulation
- Counters obstructive effect of damp and humidity
- Warms against the cold
- Strengthens the lungs

N.B. Mild aromatic herbs and spices are just right for Britain, stimulating and moving the gut without irritating it.

Using flavours to create a strong, health-giving diet for you

Seasonal weather changes are a particularly British preoccupation and climate change means that this annual cycle is less predictable than it used to be. Our most fickle of climates demands a special sort of adaptability and intelligence. That said, shielded by modern technology, we are increasingly losing our ability to respond to what the weather throws at us, and we need to retrieve it.

Adapting diet for climate

Since sweet and salty/savoury are a more or less constant part of every meal, they tend to vary little. We should eat more sweet, bland staples in winter – such as barley, chicken, potatoes, carrots and parsnips – as our calorific requirement rises, but that's about it. It's the other three flavours – sour, bitter and spicy aromatics – that are the main tastes to consider in terms of variation and adaptability.

Bitterness and spicy aromatics constantly stimulate motility to counter the dietary inhibition of cold and damp. Meanwhile, sour helps to cut through and break down the rich food that we need in the relatively cold autumn, winter and spring, and, on current climatic form, much of the summer too!

This means that a healthy British diet should be a mix of at least four of the five flavours, and as the weather gets more challenging, the flavours should get more intense. A good winter dish, such as a stew or casserole, might easily include components that are strong in all five flavours; for example, parsnip, carrot, barley or potato (sweet); beef, stock, a fermented condiment such as Worcester sauce and seasoning (salty/savoury); juniper berry, rosemary, seasonal greens and parsley (bitter); black pepper, paprika and oregano (spicy and aromatic); and tomato, vinegar, wine, cider or a pickle accompaniment (sour).

This may sound complex, but don't be put off. Most traditional dishes have a similar composition and include the three most important flavours: sour, bitter and aromatic. Responding to changes in climate is easy. First, you need to know the flavour-based characteristics of a wide range of ingredients: meat, fish, vegetables, pulses, oils, spices, herbs, nuts and fruits (see the Short Guide to Herbs, Spices and Medicinal Foods, Chapter 9). You also need to recognise the overall properties of the dishes that they constitute, from pancakes to chicken soup (see Recipes). Then you need to choose the right recipe for your circumstances, and increase or diminish the amount of each flavour according to your needs.[27]

If it gets colder, you should eat richer foods like meat or fish, and plant fats such as hemp or olive oil. You should also increase the sour accompaniment (such as pickles) to help digestion of the fats.

Consuming more aromatic spices will warm the body and stimulate circulation. In wet weather, we need to eat more aromatic spices and bitterness to stimulate motility in the gut.

However, the spicy diet for cold and damp weather needs to be balanced with cooling and refreshing flavours so that the gut does not get irritated.

To achieve this, you need bitter and sour ingredients – spinach and yoghurt in curries, for example, or pickles, tomatoes, white wine or vinegar in chilli con carne. Similarly, you should eat lighter food such as stir-fries and salads that contain more sour and bitter ingredients to cool and refresh the body when the weather is very hot.

Playing with flavours in this way is a simple principle. And once you have been practising it for a while – do use the recipes at the back of the book – you will find you opt for the right sort of dish almost instinctively.

The diagram opposite summarises the individual actions

---

27 You can find more information about combining flavours in the Recipes section of this book, which includes a range of dishes with commentaries and suggested variations on each one

of these three key flavours and how they act in combination, either as pairs or all together:

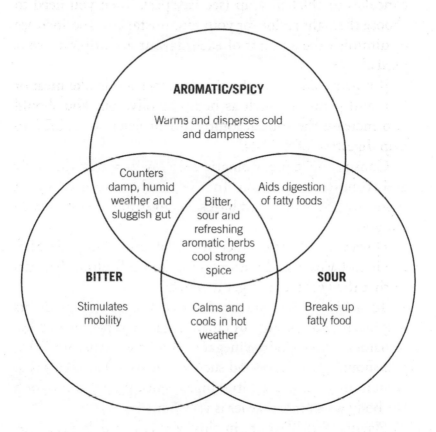

AROMATIC/SPICY

Warms and disperses cold and dampness

Counters damp, humid weather and sluggish gut

Aids digestion of fatty foods

Bitter, sour and refreshing aromatic herbs cool strong spice

BITTER

Stimulates mobility

Calms and cools in hot weather

SOUR

Breaks up fatty food

The principles of food analysis can be applied not only to individual ingredients but also to whole dishes, like the ones found in the Recipes section of this book. Here are some examples:

Climate type	Food type	Simple recipes	Average recipes	More complex recipes
Cold and damp	Rich and spicy, with a little sour and bitter to cut through the richness	Chestnut soup p.218 Spicy scrambled eggs p.230	Kedgeree p. 242 Sausage casserole p.248	Boiled ham hocks with pease pudding p.252 Slow-roasted lamb and harissa p.267
Cold and dry	Rich and aromatic	Mushroom risotto p.224 Tuna, fennel and bean salad p.232	Aromatic mussels with cider and bacon p.236 Lemon chicken p.244	Cassoulet p. 255 Chicken chasseur p.258
Hot and humid	Light, spicy and bitter	Spicy chicken broth with noodles p.222 Baked fish with herbs p.216	Salmon and caper fish cakes p.246 Spicy stir fry p.238	Chicken curry p.260 Dal p.262
Hot and dry (rare in our climate!)	Light, sour and bitter	Aromatic chicken broth with noodles p.222 Nasturtium, chicken and pesto salad p.226	Ceviche p.240 Basic stir fry p.238	Falafel p.265 Grilled or barbecued sardines with salsa p.250

Adapting diet for lifestyle and circumstance

Most of us have demanding and stressful lifestyles. I'm sure that I'm not alone in finding combining work and young children distinctly tiring. Lack of sleep, illness, accidents and bereavement all have the same debilitating effect.

Acknowledging these issues is one thing; knowing how to adapt one's diet accordingly is another. But, as we saw with mitigating against the effects of climate above, adaptation is relatively easy once you understand the principles. Most of the time we need a steady rhythmic sustenance, but there are occasions when we need to be super-charged and others when we need to be gently nurtured. For example, when you are under great physical or emotional strain, there is a need for a light, naturally sweet and digestible food such as chicken soup with barley.

Here are some other examples:

Condition	Food type	Recipe examples
Convalescence	Light, gently aromatic food	Chicken broth with noodles p.220
Tired/worn out	Regular small amounts of richer food, more heavily spiced On a foundation of blander easily digested food	Boiled ham hocks with pease pudding p.252 Pancakes p. 228, potato salad p.234, chestnut soup p.218 ... and lots of sleep!
Stressed/anxious	Light and easy to digest food with a balance of all the flavours	Lemon chicken p.244

Also take a look at the Short Guide to Herbs, Spices and Medicinal Foods (Chapter 9) for specifically calming foods (fennel, p.197-8, and rosemary, p.194 are good examples)

In China there are whole libraries devoted to foods and recipes for every imaginable circumstance and human condition. These libraries are arguably the world's greatest repository of nutritional literature; no stone is left unturned and the range of described ingredients is massive, including many that would be considered exotic at the least, and quite wacky by some. Of most interest to us, however, is the fact that much of the writing is based on an understanding of flavour.

There is a saying in China that if you see an old woman rushing up the street with a chicken under her arm, a baby has just been born. The Chinese appreciate that the best way for a woman to recover from childbirth is to eat chicken stew. When my first child was born, the best thing on offer on the maternity ward menu was plain pasta shells and cold tuna. Keen to give my wife something warm and sustaining, I dashed home (a little bleary-eyed) and got some rice-wine-fried chicken with ginger and turmeric. This strategy for recovery from childbirth is not the norm in Britain today; yet we certainly once had the same sensitivity and would have it still if we were all our own nutritionists.

The knowledge that you need for crucial nutritional adaptability is at your fingertips. The Short Guide to Herbs, Spices and Medicinal Foods (Chapter 9) is your best resource when exploiting the flavour principle. It is a reference for understanding flavour and adapting recipes to your needs, either through adding more of what you need, or identifying foods that you can definitely do without!

Don't forget the value of condiments (like those in the

Recipes section). These are great for enhancing a dish, as well as quickly modifying a dish that is already cooked.

SUMMARY

- Weather and environment affect health and well-being. Use the table and chart (pp. 93-95) to work out what sort of flavours and dishes you should be eating at any particular time.

- Dietary strategies exist for conditions such as fatigue, convalescence and emotional stress. See the recommendations in the chart on pp. 95-6. The index has some entries for specific areas such as "bowel", "stomach" and "lungs". (There are also now a number of British websites for seasonal foods, food groups and recipes that can be adapted for your needs.[28])

- Complex situations such as pregnancy require much more detailed dietary rationales and input; these are beyond the scope of this book, as are specific strategies for medical conditions. If you suffer from an illness, seek the help of an appropriately qualified health professional.

---

28 For example BBC Food, River Cottage and www.eattheseasons.co.uk

5.

How to Put Together, and Eat, a Healthy Meal

In the previous section, I focused on the understanding of flavour to facilitate choice and adaptation of recipes for a healthy diet. Recipes are incredibly useful tools in this respect as they represent the bigger picture in terms of combinations of foods and the construction of dishes and meals. They are also a great way to learn to cook, providing the kind of structure that is a perfect helping hand as we develop confidence in the kitchen.

In this age of the celebrity chef, we are arguably more familiar with recipes and recipe books than ever before – almost overwhelmingly so. You can hardly turn on the TV these days without being enticed by the best new broad bean and ricotta bruschetta.

You'd be forgiven for thinking they were a modern invention. But recipes have a long history. Indeed, they are as old as written language itself. The earliest Chinese treatise is said to be the *Shen Nong Ben Cao*, a result of the legendary emperor Shen Nong (which translates as the "Divine Farmer") tasting and classifying the actions of hundreds of foods around 5000 years ago. The resulting Chinese *materia medica* is massive, including over 5000 different species and mineral substances, and the Chinese diet is extraordinarily diverse. They also learnt a lot about toxicity: I'm afraid to say that a few of the tasters didn't make it!

In Britain we don't have such an extensive historical nutritional literature, but we do at least have some significant recipe books written over the last millennium. Of particular interest to academics are domestically generated handwritten notebooks of recipes, often embellished over generations. These include cooking tips, recipes, medicinal advice and formulas for medicaments like those found in the papers of Elizabeth Freke (1641–1714).[29]

This material, however, was inevitably accessible only to the literate, which in the pre-Victorian eras tended not to include the rural poor and urban working classes. So in fact domestic papers and published texts probably represent the tip of the iceberg in terms of the knowledge and traditions of British people. More recently, in early and mid-Victorian times, there were more recipe books available specifically for the poor and working class, such as Alexis Soyer's *Soyer's Charitable Cookery* and *Shilling Cookery for the People*.

And then there were the justly famous ones, such as Eliza Acton's *Modern Cookery* and *Mrs Beeton's Book of Household Management*. Actually, as many critics have pointed out, many of Mrs Beeton's recipes were not just impractical, they were revolting – mushy vegetables boiled to oblivion – and sometimes, as Clarissa Dickson Wright demonstrates in her *History of English Food*, positively poisonous. (Reheated lobster, anyone?)

What you realise, as you look more closely, is that these famous Victorian cookbooks were as much about aspiration and fantasy as they were about practice. Many of the recipes weren't expected to be cooked – just like many of the ones in books today. The difference is that, unlike today,

29 Leong E (2008). Making Medicines in the Early Modern Household. *Bulletin of the History of Medicine* 82: 145–168

they were beyond the reach of the working classes, who instead depended largely for information on the preparation of their food on oral traditions and lessons from their forebears.

For a really good health-promoting diet, it is fine in principle to adapt the celebrity cookbooks, but we should always work on a foundation similar to the mid-Victorian working-class diet, and modern traditional diets such as that practised by the Japanese.

And, rather than focus slavishly on what's been written down, we should learn the set of dietary principles embodied in the understanding of flavour, and use these to build our own impromptu recipes, as well as to adapt ones that already exist.

Creating meals using the flavour principle

Using flavours to create a healthy meal is remarkably simple. Balance is the key, and to achieve balance we have to approach the flavours one by one.

So we start with a staple, which is typically sweet and bland, but can be savoury. Then add salty/savoury flavour enhancers and finish with the appropriate balance of bitter, sour, spice and aromatics according to climate and lifestyle.

Start with a staple – sweet and bland

Staples are the most fundamental of foods, the foundations on which all dishes and diets are built, providing starchy calories that fuel us in our day-to-day activities.

They vary throughout the world – much Okinawan dietary value is said to be down to their use of the sweet potato, while the rest of Asia largely depends on rice, millet and wheat, which is turned into noodles and buns. Millet is eaten in parts of Africa, manioc and plantain in the Amazon basin and the Caribbean, and maize in Central America. The mid-Victorian working class depended on oats, wheat, rye and barley, whilst rice and potatoes were also popular. The Irish, meanwhile, famously depended on potatoes in this period, and the consequences were disastrous when their crops were repeatedly struck by blight.

Ireland, like the rest of the Western world, now consumes prodigious quantities of wheat, in marked contrast to the past, when it was primarily used in bread and pastry. For the mid-Victorian working class, wheat bread *was* important, but expensive, and a wide range of other foods, from starchy vegetables to oysters, were also used as staples to bulk out their diets.

In other words, because of today's large-scale wheat consumption, there is a shocking lack of variety in the staples eaten in modern non-traditional diets.

Wheat

Wheat is a popular grain because modern varieties are easily grown, modern distribution has made it relatively cheap and, due to its high gluten content, it is a doddle to process industrially.

Gluten is a sticky, stretchy protein that forms when wheat is processed. It helps food products

---

pass through processing machines very easily, trapping air and facilitating efficient bread and pastry production.

However, the very properties that make gluten so machine-friendly make it particularly digestion-unfriendly. Our enzymes and symbionts find it very hard to break down; so wheat, with its high gluten levels, is a staple that inhibits rather than promotes digestion. People with Coeliac's disease (gluten enteropathy) have a total intolerance to gluten and cannot eat any products containing wheat. And yet despite the basic digestive stubbornness of wheat, it is not uncommon for us to use wheat as the staple for all three of our daily meals; cereal or toast for breakfast, a sandwich for lunch and pasta, a pie or pizza for supper.

The effect of so much wheat in our diets is to slow us down – indeed, in traditional medicine it is used as a mild sedative and calmant – an effect that is not only undesirable but has resulted in epic levels of constipation. This, combined with our modern inactive lifestyles, means that we aren't doing enough to stimulate healthy motility. Little exercise and a wheat-heavy diet make for an unhappy gut – a balance we need to compensate for when devising our diet.

How did the mid-Victorians manage to eat bread and also maintain a healthy gut? This is a mystery that can be solved by studying the difference between the bread they ate and the mass-produced loaves we commonly consume.

A brief history of bread

The first difference between mid-Victorian bread and today's bread was that the mid-Victorians made their loaves from wholegrain flour. White flour was still expensive in those days and so the working class ate bread made from unrefined flour that included both the highly nutritious bran and germ. Ironically, this resulted in wholegrain bread being deemed a "poor man's food" and therefore undesirable. So when in the late nineteenth century more and more cheap white flour was imported from North American mills, the quality of British bread plummeted as people opted to eat the snowy white loaves that generations of their forebears had aspired to, but never been able to afford. The result was a now familiar decline in the nation's health to the extent that vigorous health campaigns were conducted in 1911 and white bread was banned entirely during the Second World War, although it was legalised again shortly afterwards.

Poor old British bread suffered another monster blow in the early 1960s, with the invention of the Chorleywood bread process, an industrial baking system that takes cheap flour with a host of chemical additives, fast-acting yeast and plenty of sugar, and turns it into something resembling bread in record time. A Chorleywood loaf is produced in under three and a half hours, from its raw ingredients to the plastic bag and pallet in which it appears. In no time at all, it's stacked neatly on the articulated lorry!

Bread is meant to be a fermented food and yet the Chorleywood process allows hardly any time for fermentation. Instead, in an extremely brief period of time, the yeast reacts violently, producing lots of gas which is trapped with the help of lots of protein (the type that obstructs digestion) and flour "improvers". The loaf is then baked into a spongy, wet, crustless approximation of what real bread should be. Incredibly – and rather disappointingly – 98% of all the bread that is baked in Britain goes through the Chorleywood process, including most of the bread that is fed to children in schools. Without wanting to sound melodramatic, this seems criminally neglectful to me.[30]

What's the alternative?

The mid-Victorians ate a bread made with low-protein wholegrain British wheat, which produced a denser, tastier loaf. This bread was twice risen, often overnight, so that the yeast had plenty of time to break down the wheat – this aided digestibility and produced a suite of fabulous extra nutrients.

Today's artisanal bakers produce a similar type of bread. It can be bought throughout Britain. Other forms of bread, which are superior to the mass-produced type are available, such as rye loaves and a range of low-gluten varieties such as bread made

---

30 Much has been written about the Chorleywood bread process. Health campaigners and traditionalists get very worked up about it! To find out more try traditional bakers' websites or baking books like *Bread* by Daniel Stevens

from spelt, an ancient form of wheat described in more detail in the Short Guide to Herbs, Spices and Medicinal Foods (Chapter 9). Sourdough loaves are also desirable; the yeasts that aid the fermentation process are more natural and digestible.

This artisan/handmade bread is expensive. The way round this problem is simply to eat less of it. Which is no bad thing. There is a current trend for nutritionists to recommend that wheat be cut out of the diet altogether for the sake of digestion. Indeed, I once did the same. Today my view is different because Britain is a nation of bread eaters. Bread lies at the core of our nutritional culture. It is, as they say, the "Staff of Life". The mid-Victorians showed us that bread can form a significant part of a healthy diet; it just has to be the *right* bread and in the right context. Essentially, because the mid-Victorians did so much more exercise than us today, the motility obstructing effect of the wheat in their bread was compensated for.

I'm not anti-bread; I'm anti-*bad* bread. My recommendation therefore is that we eat healthy artisanal bread and home-bake to cut costs, just like they did in the old days. And, of course, we should be doing more exercise, because regardless of the quality of the bread that we eat, due to the nature and quality of its proteins, wheat is a rich staple and it requires extra help to move and be digested.

Fortunately, other staples are much lighter and therefore extremely good for digestion. They should form the basis of the British diet. This greater digestibility can be due to a variety of reasons; they might have just the right amount of fibre, for example, and the right sorts of proteins and fats to stimulate and facilitate motility, or their sugars and starches may be spot on for the nourishment of our symbiotic bacteria. In most cases it's a mix of all three of these factors. With this principle of staples that support, nourish and strengthen digestion in mind, we can build a list of staples that are ideal for a healthy diet.

Grains	Vegetables	Animal Products	Beans (well cooked!)
Barley	Carrot	Beef/Lamb/	Aduki
Buckwheat	Leek	Chicken broth	Bean sprouts
Corn	Onion (well	Chicken	Haricot
Millet	cooked)	Cod/Haddock	Hyacinth
Oats	Parsnip	Plaice	Kidney
Rice	Pumpkin	Turkey	Lentils
Rye	Sweet Potato/		Split peas
	Yam		
	Turnip		

Most of the foods on this list are not considered exotic today. Indeed, as we know, the mid-Victorians depended on many of the same foods to build and maintain their health; nearly all the foods are starchy in nature and provided bulk and sustenance, fibre and a wide range of nutrients to give energy and satiety and get people through the demands of their working days. If our modern diets were constructed in the same way, we would be nourished and invigorated and would not have a tendency to put on weight.

It is worth noting that some meats, fish, beans and broths are included as staples; they were and still are used to bulk out traditional diets. They are also compatible with (healthy) modern weight-loss regimes, thus indicating a strong correlation between traditional approaches such as the mid-Victorian diet and modern protocols that help to lose weight without damaging health. I expand on this in Chapter 8.

In dietary terms, the bogey foods, the foods that are most likely to make us fat, cause diabetes and damage hearts and blood vessels in modern-day Britain, are refined sugar, refined wheat products (including Chorleywood bread) and cheap industrially processed fat.

None of these make it onto the list of Be Your Own Nutritionist staples!

If you follow the principle of using the recommended staples as a foundation for your meal, without eating too much meat or bread, then you have taken a vital step towards long-lasting health and a consistent, healthy weight.

Red meat – friend or foe?

Fresh red meat is definitely a nutritional friend! This nutritious food is and always has been a most valued component of traditional diets, and yet today it is consistently vilified as a dietary villain by medics, dieticians, politicians and fadists.

Why? As Dr John Briffa explains in his book *Escape the Diet Trap*, and also in his assessment of the most recent research on his blog, the view of red meat as disease-causing relies on imprecise epidemiological data. Decisions to exclude entire nutritional categories such as fresh red meat cannot be based on such epidemiological studies, because they cannot elucidate direct causal relationships. We can be sure that there is currently no good evidence linking fresh red meat to heart disease or cancer, for example. Indeed, there is really good evidence suggesting the opposite; fresh red meat is health-enhancing, as we have seen in the mid-Victorian case.

So what should we avoid meat-wise? First look out for the product of ropey agriculture. Animals raised predominantly on grain will have higher levels of omega 6 fats, which we know are linked to heart disease and cancer. Such animals also tend to be given antibiotics and other damaging drugs routinely.

The evidence linking industrially processed meat to cancer is also strong. Such products are packed with preservatives and other pathogenic chemicals, so eat your meat fresh rather than relying on the cheapest supermarket snags!

Build on the staple – salty and savoury

Once you have established the staple(s) in your dish, it is time to choose your salty/savoury component. There is a wide range of options, apart from the addition of refined salt itself, which I'm not encouraging.

The salty/savoury flavour component of a meal is important – it adds depth, stimulates appetite and secretion, and enhances the other flavours. Particularly fascinating in this respect is the "sixth flavour" umami, which I have included under the salty/savoury "umbrella".

Our greatest exposure to umami is through industrially produced monosodium glutamate (MSG, or E621 as

it appears on the packet), which is added to most processed foods as a cheap, possibly addictive, flavour enhancer.
Consumption of this chemical is not desirable as it bumps
up our sodium levels and consequently our blood pressure;
it *may* cause other disease and *could* be neurotoxic – there's
a scientific debate raging on this front, so you'll have to
make your own mind up on the subject!

Suffice it to say that, in health terms, industrially
produced MSG is a dirty also-ran when we compare it with
traditional, health-enhancing, umami-rich alternatives,
such as seaweed and fermented foods.

Seaweed

This is a fast-emerging superfood and one of the
main dietary reasons why the Japanese live so long.
It's delicious and was once widely eaten in Britain
too. Today the Welsh still enjoy their laverbread,
but edible seaweed lines all of Britain's shores and
needs to make something of a comeback.

N.B. Be aware that if you have a thyroid condition
you may need to exclude seaweed from you diet due
to its iodine content.

Fermented foods

These are also often umami-rich and vital as part
of a healthy diet; indeed, Weston Price identified
fermented foods as common to all of the world's
truly sustaining traditional diets. A great way to
include these foods in your diet is through sauces

such as anchovy sauce, Worcester sauce, mushroom ketchup and brown sauce (traditionally produced – not the mass-produced stuff).

Fermented sauces used to be very popular in Britain, especially in the Victorian era when there was a significant increase in the variety of both homemade and branded products. They are not at all hard to make. As an illustration, I like Clarissa Dickson Wright's description of how she made her own brown sauce.[31]

"I also once made a batch of sauce myself which essentially consisted of anchovies, garlic, horseradish and various other spices, and which I put in one of those large glass jars that you see in old fashioned sweet shops. At first it was revolting. After six months it was quite nice. After a year it was delicious."

Legend has it that Worcester sauce was originally intended as a curry sauce. It lay forgotten in a basement for several years before it was tasted and found to be delectable.

I am indebted to my grandmother, who kindly forgot about a number of chutneys, sauces and condiments, which were discovered in her garage several years later. They were treacly, mellow and delightful. Ten years on from that and we were still eating them.

It seems incredible that we've forgotten the importance of fermented sauces to nutrition in spite of their central place in traditional diets around the world. Consider the various Asian versions: soy sauce, fish sauce, shrimp paste, miso, black bean sauce and oyster

---

31 *A History of British Food* p369

sauce, among others. In many ways, choosing the savoury component of a meal is the most exciting bit.

Use savoury products like anchovy sauce, mushroom ketchup, Worcester sauce and fish sauce in your cooking and you will massively enhance its flavour and nutritional content – and you will have little or no need to add salt. Or how about using some good-quality bouillon or an organic stock cube instead?

If you really must add salt to your food, I would suggest you do what the mid-Victorians did, which is to pop a little bit of sea salt on the edge of your plate to use as and when you need it.

Add sour, bitter, spicy and aromatic

The sweet and salty/savoury flavours lay the foundations of a meal. We now need to add the other three flavours – sour, bitter and spicy/aromatic.

Using the sour, bitter and spicy/aromatic flavours is essentially *diagnostic,* and this is where you can truly become your own nutritionist. It's up to you to look at the season, the weather, what food is available, and to see how you feel within yourself, and eat accordingly; almost inevitably, regardless of what foods you choose, you will end up using all three of these flavours in different proportions, according to circumstance.

To illustrate the point, I would like to describe how my weekly working lunch turns out in different seasons with different weather, and according to how I am feeling within myself, based on one simple ingredient – mackerel.

Mackerel for lunch

Here's the scene: I work in my own house and have access to a proper kitchen. I *always* take an hour for lunch, which gives me 25 minutes cooking time, 25 minutes to eat and ten minutes for chat, tea or to accommodate my two o' clock client if he or she arrives early. Ingredients are readily available – I grow my own veg, the local organic farm sells me produce and local shops are easily accessible. So in a typical working day I tend to have everything at my fingertips to put together a good meal in a short space of time.

Starting with the staples, I choose from rice, potatoes, pasta, noodles, bulgar wheat and barley couscous. I very rarely eat bread during a working day as this slows me down.

To the staple I generally add steamed veg, which varies according to the season. Right now it's late autumn so that means pumpkin, kale, cabbage, carrots, and I will continue with these throughout the winter. Before the first frosts there was the usual early autumn glut – courgettes, squash, beans and green leaves – which carried on from late spring into summer. This means that over the course of a year I eat a huge range of vegetables, mostly (lightly) cooked.

Now to the mackerel fillets. This fish is cheap and easily frozen so it doesn't necessarily have to be bought on the day to become part of a quick and nutritious meal.

Mackerel is an oily fish and it is rich, so it must be combined with sour and aromatic flavours for digestibility. The most basic way to cook it therefore is to fry it in olive oil and/or butter and add lemon juice and black pepper. More fun is to fry it with some paprika and then add the lemon juice. I often cook it in this basic way in the summer. It takes less than five minutes.

As the weather gets colder and wetter in autumn, winter

and spring, and also if I am feeling tired, it is nice to have a bit of a sauce with the fish. The meal is then richer and more flavoursome. Two simple ways to achieve this are by poaching it in white wine (sour),[32] coconut milk or a chicken or fish stock (savoury). To these can be added finely chopped shallot (aromatic), juniper berries (bitter), black peppercorns (spicy) and lemon zest (bitter and aromatic). The poaching liquid then becomes the sauce to be poured over the fish and the staple. Another advantage of this method is that it is easy to cook whole fish with heads on: this is much more nutritious as some of the goodness of the bones and the head passes into the sauce. Cooking whole fish this way takes 10-15 minutes, while frying or poaching fillets takes 2-5 minutes.[33]

To my fish and veg I normally add a nice little something like pickled capers or nasturtium seeds (sour and aromatic), olives (aromatic, salty/savoury, sweet and bitter depending on the olive) or sun-dried toma-toes. Sometimes I might have a couple of nasturtium flowers straight off the plant (bitter and aromatic). These grow throughout most of the summer and autumn. Typically, I also make a dressing to have on the vegeta-bles, combining an oil from olive, hemp or rapeseed, a little mustard (spicy and aromatic), soy sauce (savoury) and cider vinegar (sour, and a West Country classic). My ethnically Chinese traditional medicine colleagues are very fond of recommending mustard to their clients

---

32 I must reassure my acupuncture clients that the alcohol is boiled off the wine as it is cooked – I never have alcohol during a working day!

33 Every now and then I end up with smoked mackerel. This is very rich and benefits from marinating in lemon juice, lemon zest and black pepper for at least 30 minutes, lightening the meat and making it much more digestible.

as it is said to stimulate the lungs to protect against our damp climate, so when the weather is damp and cold I add more mustard and oil to make the meal richer and more spicy and aromatic. In summer I add more vinegar to lighten the meal and make it more refreshing. In summer I also tend to add more chopped, fresh, refreshing leafy herbs such as coriander and parsley (aromatic).

Pudding

And what about pudding? In summer and early autumn, fruit stewed with ginger (or stem ginger) and cinnamon is wonderfully nourishing. Otherwise walnuts (bitter) and honey (I have a walnut tree in my garden), chestnuts (sweet) and almonds (bitter and slightly aromatic) are delicious, especially in autumn, winter and early spring. And I often have some 73% dark chocolate (bitter), which sounds indulgent but it's pure medicine to me.

I often eat quite a lot at lunchtime; indeed I'm known as a big eater, and I always have to go straight back to work in a busy clinic. But, because the meal is balanced, I never feel tired or troubled by indigestion. Food like this is so much easier to deal with, the keys being the achievement of balance through flavour, and taking a little time to prepare and cook.

***

So now let's look at what my diet during a typical day might look like:

A Typical Day's Menu

Breakfast	Eat hot food and definitely no breakfast cereal! Here are some ideas: Spicy scrambled eggs (p. 230) Pancakes (p. 228) Poached egg, black pudding, toast and butter with a sprinkle of paprika Good bread/toast and butter and marmalade Spiced stewed fruit with homemade muesli/porridge. Try cooking porridge with ginger and/or cinnamon Soup/broth with noodles Bubble and squeak with spring onion and black pepper
Lunch	Leftovers – a great strategy is always to cook double the amount the night before or to have a cook-up at the weekend so there are plenty of leftovers in the fridge or freezer Eat at home – by cooking a quick meal as I described earlier (p. 112) Eat out – by choosing digestion-friendly providers. In summer noodle bars often do the trick. In winter it is a case of finding good quality, hearty food wherever it is sensibly priced. If you have a work canteen, show the chef this book!
Supper	This is when we tend to have the most time to cook, and to enjoy cooked food. So start with the recipes in this book then branch out. Just think flavour and adaptability. And remember to cook extra so that you can freeze portions for kids and busy times, and keep some in the fridge for tomorrow's lunch.

Time to Cook

The modern approach to cooking would be unrecognisable to our ancestors. How things have changed! In the last 50 years the daily time spent cooking in the UK has more or less *halved*. But, like all of life's great skills, to be good at cooking we have to take the time to practise recognition of food and its value, and develop *connection*, through smells, textures, colour and taste.

These values were recognised in traditional nutritional approaches. In centuries past, cooking had greater significance than just sticking a pan on a burner. Instead, it was revered as a series of complex, intriguing and delightful processes. So we really should see cooking not just as a way of heating our food, but as a form of *preparation*, or even the first stage of digestion.

Preparation **is** cooking

Chopping

The ancient Chinese recognised the essential importance of food preparation by referring to cooking as *ge peng* – literally translated as "cut and cook". Hence chopping has long been approached by the Chinese with the same diligent vigour and passion as any other kitchen craft; while there are literally hundreds of cooking methods throughout China, and there are just as many ways of chopping the ingredients.

Fuchsia Dunlop, who trained as a chef in Sichuan, illustrates this attention to detail in her book *Shark's Fin and Sichuan Pepper: A Sweet-Sour Memoir of Eating in China*. Among other skills she was taught to chop in myriad different ways – "domino" slices, "ox-tongue" slices, "chopstick" strips, "horse" ears, "thumbnail" slices, "eyebrows", "fish-eye" spring onions, "rice grains", cubes, "blossoming" spring onions, "phoenix" tails and "silver-needle" slivers.

Our healthy diet doesn't require skill of this magnitude, but it does require just a little bit of *time*. Time to choose great ingredients, time to cut them up carefully, not just to make them look attractive but to release flavours, and time to prepare them in other ways.

Marinating

Marinating (like the smoked mackerel with lemon juice that I have already mentioned) is an example of a key preparation method. Marinades tend to be acidic, setting up a pre-digestion process in which the acids start to break down the complex molecules of the food. This is a form of pre-digestion that is particularly helpful for tough and rich foods; the marinating gives our digestion a valuable helping hand. It also introduces flavours to a dish early on, giving them a chance to meld and mature.

The digestive effect of marinating can be so powerful that some dishes, such as the Mexican ceviche (see Recipes section), require no heating at all, the lime juice and spices making the fish tender enough to be eaten raw. Pickled herring, that was once consumed in Britain and is still widely consumed in Scandinavian countries, is based on the same principle. Likewise, the mid-Victorians ate a lot of pickled foods such as whelks, mussels and cockles as street food. These shellfish tended to be cooked before they were brined and pickled; however, the effect of the vinegar will still have helped digestibility.

Cooking **is** essential

Humans and hominids have been cooking, or "thermally processing" food for over a million years. We absolutely depend on heating up our food to be healthy, and so does every major traditional dietary culture in the world. Cooking food takes the complex molecules that make up food structure and breaks them down. The cellulose packaging and fibrous scaffold of plant food is broken apart so that we can easily access the nutrients within, and soluble fibre, vital for motility, is generated. In animal foods, the structural proteins like collagen are broken down to form soluble proteins such as gelatin. Gelatin is a wonderfully nourishing nutrient that is specifically created by cooking. In addition to making food digestible, cooking helps flavours in combinations of ingredients to interact, develop and mellow. Similarly, nutrients from different foods intermingle and react, enhancing each other's actions, an effect known as synergism.

As a general rule, the more tough and fibrous a food is, the more we need to cook it. Foods such as beans, some root vegetables and cheap cuts of meat like shin of beef or oxtail, lend themselves to gentle, slow cooking in soups, stews and casseroles, and, once they have been cooked like this, they become extremely nutritious. In other words, the right cooking method turns cheap food into some of the most healthy – the best food that money can buy. Of course, this kind of long cooking requires some planning. Slow cookers, hay boxes and the like are great in this respect, as are warming ovens that can be used to cook food over several hours. When I'm at work I will happily put a stock, tough vegetables, beans or cheap cuts of meat on a very low burner in the morning while I get on with other things.

By contrast, when it comes to lighter foods like grains, potatoes and whole fish, and even lighter foods like leafy greens and chicken and fish fillets, we can ease the overall intensity of the cooking, from baking to boiling to steaming to stir-frying, to maintain freshness and nutrient content without compromising the taste of the food.

So the method that we use to cook our food is important in terms of health and the availability of nutrients. There is a balance to be struck. Some foods actually become more nutritious the longer that they are cooked, most notably bone stocks and tough cuts of meat. Dried beans have to be cooked for a long time to be edible and other tough plant material such as kale is much more palatable if it has been cooked well.

Other foods are more nutritious with less cooking, for example, vitamin C which is thermally degradable – we have to cook plant foods to get to more of the nutrients from them, but if we cook them too much we will destroy a lot of the goodness. Therefore, a little bit of cooking can go a long way; just five minutes of steaming or stir-frying makes a big difference.

The cooking method is also important, as nutrients may leach into the cooking water, or be destroyed at high temperatures. Boiling leaches more than steaming, although this becomes incidental if cooking water is used in a sauce or retained for use in a bone stock. However, both these water-based methods are preferable to baking and roasting, which involve temperatures higher than the boiling point of water: an important difference, since when food is cooked at a temperature above 100°C, cancer-causing chemicals are formed.

The mid-Victorian experience is informative in this respect. Because fuel was expensive, the working class typically had no ovens and cooked at lower temperatures even when grilling or frying, hence fewer cancer-causing mutagens were formed and fewer nutrients were destroyed. These methods bear a remarkable similarity to those used by the Chinese and Japanese today, who mostly boil, steam and stir-fry over a burner. And the domestic Chinese have no ovens, relying on a wok and a few bamboo steaming trays, just like the working-class mid-Victorians, who rarely possessed more than a kettle, a saucepan and a skillet.

Seasonal cooking

How you cook your food affects its qualities, and this means that different methods are more suited to different seasons:

- *Late autumn, winter, early spring* – rich food is needed for cold weather. Soups, stews and casseroles can be rich and easy to digest. Baking and roasting concentrate food to make it richer but harder to digest; they shouldn't be overused as high heat can form cancer-causing chemicals
- *Late spring, early summer* – mix bakes, stews and soups with lighter, moister steamed and boiled foods. The occasional well-dressed salad is fine
- *Hot summer* – steamed and stir-fried food predominates, with some dressed salads. Use offal and bones for light soups, broths, stews, dips and patés
- *Early autumn* – anything goes. The weather is changeable and there is a glut of vegetables and fruit. An Indian summer means more stir-fries, steamed veg and light grilling and braising. Early storms and rain mean soup, stews, casseroles and bakes.

Microwaving

The best thing that you can do with your microwave oven is take it to the tip and throw it away. Microwaves destroy a breathtaking proportion of the nutrients in food as the microwaves penetrate deep and blow them apart.[34] Microwaving also produces cancer-causing substances,[35] and, when cooking with plastic, so-called oestrogenic or hormone-mimicking chemicals[36] which have been linked to a range of diseases and conditions including obesity, cancer, polycystic ovarian syndrome (PCOS) and endometriosis. These devices have no place in our homes.

Time to eat

Eating well depends entirely on good food and the promotion of parasympathetic nervous system function. In short, we should be steady and unflustered when we eat.

This book is all about good food, but just as important is the environment that you choose or create to eat it in. So, stay calm, avoid rushing, enjoy yourself, seek good company and avoid intense distraction. Then you'll be able to relax and focus on the food itself and give the digestive process the respect that it deserves.

---

34 Vallejo F *et al.* (2003). Phenolic compound contents in edible parts of broccoli inflorescences after domestic cooking. *Journal of the Science of Food and Agriculture* 83 (14), pp1511-1516

35 Lee L (1989). Health effects of microwave radiation – microwave ovens. Lancet, December 9

36 Yang CW *et al.* (2011). Most plastic products release estrogenic chemicals: a potential health problem that can be solved. *Environmental Health Perspectives* 119:989-996. http://dx.doi.org/10.1289/ehp.1003220

Eating at home

In this context, *setting up* the environment for a meal is always important, a process that the French, Chinese and other healthy eating cultures have fiercely protected into modern times, and that has been notably eroded in modern Britain. As many as half of British households no longer use a dining table or eat daily family meals, and in 2011, 46% of all home meals were eaten alone, despite the fact that other family members were often around.[37]

The thought of such deterioration of values has the French choking on their *escargots à la bourguignonne*!

Traditional, healthy, dietary cultures, such as those in the Mediterranean, still have a daily devotion to ritual. The dining table has pride of place, and before the meal, places are set with proper cutlery, crockery and napkins. Children often have their own place-mats, interesting and colourful knives, forks, spoons, plates and bowls to foster their interest in food. Anticipation, interest and appetite are built with aperitifs. And in France at least, alcohol tends to have a relaxing effect at this stage, an effect that is also fiercely protected; according to French law all alcohol is banned while employees are at work... with the exception of wine, beer, pear cider and apple cider!

The ritual and relaxation continues when the meal arrives, as time is devoted to eating. Food is typically complimented and discussed and conversation continues in a lively and humorous atmosphere.

It is no exaggeration to describe French family meals in this way, and my experience of dining with Chinese families is the same. With one exception: in China *sometimes* the TV is on during meals. But unlike in Britain, the TV is nearly always ignored. This may be a product of the Chinese culture of *re nao* which literally translates as "hot noise", but

37 Family Food Panel survey (2011)

more broadly means a lively, happy or stimulating atmosphere that is desirable for the enjoyment of food. In other words, the Chinese have a culture that uses noise to relax, in contrast to the West. So if the TV is on they are much better than weare at tuning out of it and focusing on their food, and each other.

Children

I rather like the French idea that post-toddler children should eat what adults eat, a strategy well described in *French Kids Eat Everything* by Karen le Billon. This is an approach that is pursued with varying degrees of success in the Cooper household! It is certainly the case that if your diet is easy to digest and adapted for season and climate, then it will benefit your children's health too.

Eating alone

As an erstwhile confirmed bachelor and sole clinical operator, I eat many a lone meal. In certain circumstances they are unavoidable, and in some, desirable. When eating alone, one cannot benefit from conversation and so other methods should be found to relax. To wit, I'm going to be a bit controversial and suggest that TV dinners can be OK. The TV can be a distraction from daily stresses and can help to settle the mind, but be careful – programmes should be edifying; after a few attempts, I'm afraid I had to stop watching *Fawlty Towers* and English cricket at mealtimes; too often I got emotionally engaged in Basil Fawlty's disasters and the endless clatter of wickets.

Eating at work

Work lunches should be eaten anywhere but at the desk or on the shop floor. This is the only way to avoid your brain being engaged by "jobs to be done". Remember: the brain and emotional centres are resource-hungry and will steal vital circulation from the gut given the chance.

To this end, it is important to turn off your phone during lunch so that you can keep your attention on food and company and away from client liaison, agendas and emails.

Time to digest

Once a meal is prepared, cooked and eaten, it is the job of our digestive system to extract the maximum benefit from the food. What our guts need is just a little time.

The principle of taking time to digest is very much at odds with our modern lifestyles. As I write this, I can virtually guarantee that there are thousands of Britons who, after cracking through their lunchtime sandwiches, are gamely attempting to continue working through a fog of fatigue; a fatigue that arises through the unavoidable splitting of their resources.

On the one hand, our unmistakably human, energy-hungry brains are ploughing through a whopping 25% of our metabolic energy. On the other, energy-hungry guts are banking on a good 30%-plus of our metabolism being made available to get on with the current, post-prandial, digestive challenge. This leaves around 40% of our energy for our limbs and the rest of our organs to function effectively so that we feel invigorated and capable: impossible!

We're left with three options in relation to our

energy "budget" and the needs of our digestive systems: work on and muddle through (illness and chronic fatigue awaits); stop eating the sandwiches and eat more digestible food (preferable); or eat great food then rest and digest (perfect).

Eating and resting

The proof is truly in the pudding as far as eating and resting are concerned. Cultures that routinely take naps after lunch are far more healthy than typical Westerners. The most studied of these populations are around the Mediterranean; the South of France, Italy, Greece, Malta, etc. Put simply, the people in these deeply traditional cultures live longer, healthier, happier lives than their stressed-out ultra-industrial counterparts to the north. This is scientifically proven to be in part due to their habit of resting after lunch.[38]

For most of us, the Anglo-Saxon lifestyle just doesn't seem to permit 30 minutes to lie down after lunch. Whether we're mums with young children, we run our own businesses or we're under constant pressure to fulfil deadlines, there just doesn't seem to be the time to stop and rest.

The tendency of Anglo-Saxon-influenced cultures to eschew the siesta is strange when we consider that some of the most productive nations on earth, China and Japan, have a deep reverence for the need to "rest and digest". So ingrained is this habit that books have been written about the amusing places that the Chinese have been caught napping: on window sills, bicycles, doorsteps and under tables. I have personally had Chinese strangers fall asleep

---

38 Trickopoulou A *et al.* (2007). Midday napping slows heart disease. *Archives of Internal Medicine* 167: 296-301.

on me on buses and trains. For the Chinese, sleep is just too important to resist using a stranger as a pillow when you're in need of a nap.

Put simply, if we take a little time to allocate *most* of our energy to digestion after a meal, then we can concentrate harder, be more energetic *and* live longer and healthier lives.

The rest-and-digest compromise

So, if we absolutely can't persuade our bosses, babies and consciences to allow us to develop this intelligent convention of resting and digestion, what do we do?

We have to find a sensible compromise.

The first compromise is to take some time, *any* time, to focus our resources on the energy-hungry process of digestion. Two minutes is better than one. Five minutes is better than two. Ten minutes is better than five. Just sit back, close your eyes, cut out the surrounding stimuli – noise, lights, people – and *digest*.

The second compromise is where this book comes in. If we're not prepared to allow our bodies time to digest, then we need to make our food more *digestible*. A working sandwich lunch is bad in this respect – preserved meats, salad and cheap mass-produced bread are extraordinarily hard to break down and absorb once we have eaten them. They sit like a lump in our stomachs, sucking the vitality away from our brains. Instead, we should be eating easy-to-digest staples, with good-quality proteins and fats, vegetables and lots of spicy, aromatic, bitter and sour flavours; all adjusted according to the needs of the dish.

Eating a well-balanced hot meal at lunchtime is not easy, when you are working in an office and reliant on local fast-food providers every day. I would suggest you bring more food in from home – though since this would probably entail reheating it in a microwave, it is worth investing in wide-necked, insulated food flasks.

In the long run, however, it is probably easier if we urge our cafés, canteens and kitchens to produce this wonderful, hot, easy-to-digest, flavourful food for us.

Perhaps, as you plough through your next insipid salad or claggy sandwich, you will consider these words from Lieutenant Hornblower as he looked up from his plate of chops and pressed half a crown into the hand of Suzie, the skinny scullery maid: "Take this, and promise me that the first chance that comes your way, the moment Mrs Mason lets you out, you'll buy yourself something to eat. Fill that wretched little belly of yours. Faggots and pease pudding, pigs' trotters, all the things you like. Promise me."[39]

Hearty, nourishing stuff indeed.

---

39 Forester, CS (1952). *Lieutenant Hornblower*

6.

The Be-Your-Own-Nutritionist Food Tower

Our understanding of flavour tells us *what* we should be eating, but not necessarily *how much* of each food.

Let's start by saying that it is unlikely that we will ever need to eat as much as the mid-Victorians did. Their activity levels were extraordinary and they needed fuel to match. The modern equivalents might be professional sportsmen and women.

But we should, as a rule of thumb, copy the *relative* amounts of food types that they ate, particularly because this mirrors the conventions of other long-living traditional societies such as the Mediterraneans and the Okinawans.

The best way to convey this rule of thumb is by constructing our own food tower, broken down into different sections to represent the balance of food groups that we should be eating, and in what proportions.

Each level represents a food group, and the area that each food group takes up on the tower is *roughly* equal to the proportion of our diet that that particular food group should occupy. This means that there is great flexibility in terms of how we eat – the tower does not portray absolute dietary rules, just guidelines. It is a moveable feast that is designed to accommodate our changing nutritional needs, and of course our uniquely British climate.

FOOD TOWER

FRESH FATS (vegetable & animal)

HERBS, SPICES & MEDICINAL FOODS

SEEDS & NUTS

FRUITS

MEAT, FISH & EGGS

GRAINS & BEANS

FRESH VEGETABLES

  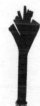

How the tower differs from pyramids

The tower is a simple visual way of showing us what proportion of our diet should be taken up by different types of foods. If we compare it with other food pyramids we can see how much more nourishing age-old, traditional diets are.

Food pyramids found on breakfast cereal boxes, for example, include far too much... breakfast cereal! These cereals are mass-produced for industrial and commercial convenience and are therefore nutritionally compromised.[40] However, they can also be found on other graphics such as the UK government's own "eatwell plate", along with dedicated sections for junk food, soda pop and Chorleywood white factory bread.[41] Such foods should not, in my opinion, be found on *any* dietary guidance for health. They were responsible for the nutritional demise of the late Victorians, as well as numerous other traditional populations (for example, the Australian Aborigines) and are the curse of our children today; they simply shouldn't have an officially sanctioned place in diet.

While government and food corporation pyramids include factory food that we should definitely be avoiding, fad diets earnestly direct us *away* from these foods towards foods that are far too extreme and may lead to eating habits that will damage health. Calorie-controlled diets, for example, tend to include far too much raw food and not enough nourishing fats.

---

40 For more information see: *Cerealizing America: The Unsweetened Story of American Breakfast Cereal* by Scott Bruce and Bill Crawford; *Eat Your Heart Out: Why the food business is bad for the planet and for your health* by Felicity Lawrence and *In Defence of Food: The Myth of Nutrition and the Pleasures of Eating* by Michael Pollan.

41 This is absolutely true at the time of writing!

Diets that encourage broader consumption of richer foods for body-fat reduction, which can form part of a healthy weight-loss regime, often fail to emphasise the importance of nutritional variety. They also have no understanding of the importance of cooking and combining these rich foods for digestibility.

This can lead to basing the diet on a limited range of foods, which can be harmful; people end up eating too much steak and chicken breast rather than whole fish, offal, marrow, bone stocks and cheap cuts that lean, healthy traditional populations have valued over millennia. As a result, many people on so called low-carb diets can risk nutritional deficiencies.

To deepen our understanding of what a balanced and nutritionally rich diet looks like, let's explore each section of the food tower in turn.

Fresh fats

There is a distinctly proud place for fats and oils in this tower: from animal fats, such as dripping, suet and butter, to plant fats, like olive oil and flax, walnut, rapeseed and sesame oils.

Fats are fundamental to health, and, as I have detailed earlier, these include not just the fats that are officially recognised as health-enhancing, such as omega 3s and monounsaturates, but also fats that have in recent decades been considered woefully unhealthy. It is beyond question that traditional diets, such as the Mediterranean diet, which government gurus, dieticians and epidemiologists are making a huge fuss about, are positively *founded* on the stuff, from the fat of free-ranging pigs, to olive oil, a wonderful aromatic, moistening and rich food in its freshest form.

In Britain, as in much of the industrialised world, our view of fat has become incredibly warped, in this bloated age of obesity, excessive consumption and cheap industrially manipulated hydrocarbons. But let it be understood: eaten in hearty moderation, good, fresh, natural fats are very good food. They fill us up, suppressing our appetites so that we don't overeat and put on weight, and they provide essential fatty acids (EFAs), vital building blocks for our cells and nervous systems. For these reasons, long-living, healthy folk all over the world depend on consuming appreciable amounts of fat for their well-being.

The animal fats that the mid-Victorians consumed, such as butter, suet, lard and their beloved beef dripping, were also truly healthy. This is because the animals then were the equivalent of today's rare breeds and were fed predominantly on pasture, rather than the grain and soy that modern industrially reared animals are given. This broadened the nutritional profile of the meat and milk, and raised levels of those all-important omega 3 EFAs.[42, 43]

The story of how fat has come to be so misunderstood in recent times is a long and complex one, involving a range of commercial, medical, cultural and political influences. The detail of this story can be found in two excellent books, Michael Pollan's *In Defence of Food: The Myth of Nutrition and the Pleasures of Eating* and Gary Taubes' *Why We Get Fat and What to Do about It*. And the conclusion of both authors is the same: don't be afraid of fat. Instead, use the

---

42 Nuernberg K *et al* (2005). Effect of a grass-based and a concentrate feeding system on meat quality characteristics and fatty acid composition of longissimus muscle in different cattle breeds. *Livestock Production Science* 94: 137–147

43 Ellis KA, Innocent D, Grove-White D, Cripps P, McLean WG (2006). Comparing the fatty acid composition of organic and conventional milk. *Journal of Dairy Science* 89: 1938–50

wisdom of traditional diets to choose from a wide range of healthy fats, staples and other foods to construct your meal and, above all, buy the best quality ingredients that you can afford. In this context, the fat component of this food tower is flexible; you can adjust the amount you eat according to your needs and lifestyle. The amount shown here could certainly be increased proportionately, with no risk to health. The important thing is to relax when it comes to fat as a food. As long as the fat isn't margarine, that is.

Saturated Fats

Contrary to the prevailing view, animal fat does not *cause* heart disease, while the omega 6 fats in margarine do[44]. There is no evidence that eating less animal fat improves health or extends our lives; in fact recent research actually links this important nutrient to well-being and happiness[45].

This importance of fat was recognised by the mid-Victorians, the traditional Chinese and other cultures. The biggest survey of hunter-gatherer diets to date has shown that 28-58% of their calories came predominantly from animal fat. They would target the fattest animals possible and preferred the fat, organs and other offal to the lean meat.[46]

44 Gilman M. *et al* (1997). Margarine intake and subsequent coronary heart disease in men. *Epidemiology* 8(2): 144-49
45 Van Oudenhove L *et al.* (2011). Fatty acid-induced gut-brain signaling attenuates neural and behavioral effects of sad emotion in humans. *Journal of Clinical Investigation* 121(8): 3094-99
46 Cordain L *et al* (2000). Plant-animal subsistence ratios and macronutrient energy estimations in worldwide hunter-gatherer diets. *American Journal of Clinical Nutrition* 71(3): 682-92

Butter

The best available evidence indicates that butter (so cherished by the mid-Victorians, and me!) does not raise heart disease levels. I adore the taste of butter, while margarine – with its water content, colouring and industrially modified oils – seems insipid. Indeed, as I mention earlier, omega 6 fats such as those found in margarine, sunflower oil and a number of other plant fats *have* been linked to heart disease among other pathologies.[47]

Herbs, spices and medicinal foods

These foods are extremely important and significantly under-represented in diets for health, for the likely reason that their biochemistry is so complex that scientists and nutritionists get their knickers in a twist when they try to understand the effects they have on the body. I deal with that problem in practice by focusing on flavour instead of chemistry.

These foods are so valuable because the vast majority of them have strong flavours and consequently strong actions. We should turn to these foods to achieve an effect in a dish, to create balance and compensate for prevailing climate, life-style or emotion. As the Chinese say, "food is medicine".

Medicinal foods without strong flavours, such as mushrooms, certain nuts, fruits and offal, cross over with other food categories in the tower but since they have such a

47 Kuipers R *et al* (2011). Saturated fat, carbohydrates and cardiovascular disease. *The Netherlands Journal of Medicine* 69 (9)

fundamental role in wellbeing, providing intense and sustaining nutrition for vibrant health and long life, I have given them their own special place in it in contrast to any other food pyramid or chart that I have ever seen.

To underline the importance of herbs, spices and medicinal foods, there is a chapter devoted to them in the book, the Short Guide to Herbs, Spices and Medicinal Foods (Chapter 9), and it provides much more information about their use in cooking.

Seeds and nuts

These are nutrient-dense and undoubtedly a major reason for the mid-Victorian working class's exceptional health. They had walnuts and chestnuts as street food and habitually gathered a wide range of nuts and seeds, including cobnuts (a type of hazelnut) when they were in season. The Chinese and Japanese also value nuts and seeds as snack foods and sources of valuable oils.

Fruit

Britain is world famous for its fruit and the mid-Victorians ate loads of it. We all know about apples, pears, blackberries, strawberries and plums, but what about the fruits that are strong in action and therefore medicinal? A few are outlined in Chapter 9 for your interest.

Most sets of food guidelines recommend more fruit than this, but I do urge caution in this respect. Fruit fibre can be very hard to break down (like bananas, especially when they are not completely ripe), tropical fruits such as pineapples and mangos can be very sugary and create digestive imbalance, and the acidity of fruits such as apples, plums and citrus in the wrong context can easily disturb the gut. For this reason, many people with IBS struggle with raw fruit, much to their frustration, as it perceived in our culture as being particularly healthy. They are suffering from a common dietary error – raw is rarely best in Britain! In digestive terms, most fruit should be eaten dried, or spiced and cooked, especially when the weather is cold and damp.

Meat, fish and eggs

This section of the tower is reasonably large to reflect its place in the working-class mid-Victorians' diet. They ate as much fish, fresh and preserved meat and eggs as they could, to the extent that any absence of these foods in their daily meals was considered a sign of poverty.

It is easy to see how this quantity of consumption is justified nutritionally in relation to seafoods. They are crammed with essential oils and minerals and make it onto just about every healthy eating chart around. Weston Price's observation was that, despite the great variety in the diets of healthy traditional cultures that he recorded, they all had a special place for seafood, no matter how far they were from the sea. Seafoods contain essential nutrients difficult to obtain from any other food. In remote land-locked countries like Mongolia, for example, the trade in dried fish and fish eggs was, and still is, considered extremely important.

By contrast, meat has had a rougher ride than fish in recent times. We seem frightened of its fat content (unjustifiably, as unbiased scientific evidence suggests) and similarly scared of its supposed link to a range of diseases, such as bowel cancer.

I think that it's important to keep things in perspective

here. Many of the studies on the association between red meat and disease are based in the USA where meat consumption is at incredible levels. They eat a large amount of industrially processed and preserved-meat products, and they are often eating animals raised in appalling conditions and fed on imbalanced and wholly unnatural diets. When this is compared to regular consumption of good amounts of fresh, non-industrially processed meat of any variety that is the product of good husbandry, the contrast could not be greater, in nutritional (as well as ethical) terms. The way that we eat meat today is not traditional. Cellophane-wrapped, broiler hen "skin-off" breasts are a far cry from the mid-Victorian diet that depended as much on offal as the more conventional cuts. Pigs' trotters, tripe, brain, kidney, liver, bone marrow, sweetbreads, belly, tongue and ear were not only regular fare, but considered delicacies. They are also the most nutritious part of the animal.

As for eggs, it is time to dispel a modern myth once and for all. In the vast majority of cases eggs *do not* raise unhealthy cholesterol levels and are not a cause of heart disease![48] In my lifetime I have seen government recommended egg consumption levels rise from seven a week to ten to fourteen, a ridiculous *volte-face* in policy that is, however, debunking the claims of shoddy science and food companies with a dubious agenda. Eggs, of course, are essentially nourishing, providing everything necessary to produce a new life in the form of a chick; and they're just as good for us too. So in a balanced diet it is absolutely fine to eat two eggs a day.

Overall then, seafoods, eggs, meat and offal are all

---

48 Herron L & Fernandez M (2004). Are the current dietary guidelines regarding egg consumption appropriate? *Journal of Nutrition* 134: 187-190

wonderful foods that add vital richness to our diets in the face of busy lives and a cold, damp climate.

This sounds like a licence for gluttony. This is not my intention; most people would agree that we need to impose some sort of limit on meat consumption, and that this limit should be based on sound, fad-free reasoning.

The anthropologist Richard Lee has observed that the proportion of hunted foods in the diets of a large number of hunter-gatherer societies varied between 20% and 45% with an average of 35%.[49] Similarly, a more recent and extensive paper summarised the diets of 229 hunter-gatherers,[50] showing that animal foods made up the bulk of the diets of the vast majority of these populations. Only 14% got more than half their calories from plant foods. All of them ate meat and an average of two-thirds of their calories came from animal sources and only one third from plants.

That these aboriginal and traditional diets were, and are, optimal for health has been demonstrated many times, not least by Weston Price.[51] Anthropologists have consistently demonstrated that hunter-gatherer and aboriginal diets were underpinned by wisdom, structure and intent; many papers have been written on the subject. And, since the proportion of meat eaten is consistent across such a large number of diets examined in these studies, they are our best available guide to how much meat we should be eating.

For our purposes Richard Lee's average of 35% is

49 Lee RB (1968) What Hunters Do for a Living, or, How to Make Out on Scarce Resources in Lee RB & Devore I (Eds) *Man the Hunter*, Chicago: Aldine

50 Cordain L *et al* (2000) Plant-Animal subsistence ratios and macronutrient energy estimations in worldwide hunter-gatherer diets. *American Journal of Clinical Nutrition* 71(3): 682-92

51 see *Nutrition and Physical Degeneration* by Weston Price (first pub 1939) and the Weston A Price Foundation (http://www.westonaprice.org)

probably right for modern Britain, since we need a constant level of richness to compensate for our climate. The bar for fish, meat and eggs on my tower represents a smaller proportion of overall diet than 35%, although some of the shortfall could be made up from the bar for fats. However, there are some key factors affecting modern Britain that could compromise this figure of 35%. First is that issue of price. There are more of us now than the hunter gatherer days or the Victorian era. We depend exclusively on agricultural land, so good quality meat is expensive and less available than it would have been to a wide-ranging hunter or hard-working artisan of the past. Second, seafoods are unsustainably fished and less available than they used to be, due to pollution and fisheries policies; remember: before toxicity and overfishing wiped out most of the oyster beds, oysters were so abundant they were known as a poor man's food.

These factors mean that, for environmental sustainability, we *need* to rely more on plant foods, in particular plant fats and foods that are rich in protein. So, take your pick on animal foods; you can feel relaxed if they make up 15-50% of your diet, although the less meat and fish that you eat then the more richness you have to make up from plant sources such as oils, nuts and seeds. And, of course, beans.

Grains and beans

Beans are the protein-rich reason that we can get away with eating less meat. Because of their protein content, beans are much more substantial and filling than other plant foods. The mid-Victorians ate loads of beans, also known as "legumes" as they're from the leguminosae family or "pulses" (from a middle English word *puls* meaning a "thick pap of meal"). For example, lentils were routinely used to thicken or bulk out soups and stews, and fresh beans were regular fare. Pulses are also a major part of Japanese and Chinese diets (bean sprouts, mung, hyacinth and aduki beans) and the Mediterranean diet (haricot, borlotti, black and broad beans, chickpeas, etc.).

I'm particularly fond of beans as many of them have important medicinal properties. For example, aduki beans have long been known to compensate for the pathogenic effects of damp climate; a number of other examples of their benefits are outlined in Chapter 9. Beans should be part of the modern British diet, with lentils found in every store cupboard. I should add the proviso that they can generate tremendous wind in the early stages of an increase in consumption levels. Soaking dried beans well, then thoroughly rinsing them and boiling them with kelp can help to reduce this effect. It is certainly essential to boil beans for a long time to deactivate poisonous lectins and enzyme inhibitors. In the early years I found boiling with kelp produced variable results; now I've eaten so many beans that I can approach big servings of pulses without fear of embarrassing results!

Grains are also important staples, although not quite as exciting in medicinal terms as beans. The properties of the most important healthy grains are outlined in Chapter 9. As I have already described, the primary role of grains is to act as staples to fill us up, although, as you will read later, if you intend to lose weight you may need to modify your grain intake.

Fresh vegetables

This is unquestionably an important part of the food tower. The bottom line is that we simply don't eat enough fresh vegetables and yet they are foods that do so much to make us tick. The medicinal properties of some vegetables are outlined in Chapter 9. See also the vegetables on the list of bitter foods (p. 87). These are definitely worth including as a priority in your diet. But otherwise we just need to get to know local veg when it is in season, grow it ourselves, head off to the greengrocer and, above all, eat the stuff.

What we shouldn't be eating

This diet for Britain is an inclusive diet. Its nourishing quality depends on its variety and adaptability. We have to *choose liberally* from the wide range of healthy foods that are available to sustain ourselves in the long term and provide obvious enjoyment from the plate. Similarly, we have to regain lost ground and *eat much more traditionally,* so that those foods that are the most nourishing, like offal and shellfish, mushrooms, beans, vegetables, nuts and wild fruits, find their way back onto our kitchen tables.

In this context, I am keen to keep the list of, in health terms at least, prohibited foods short. Here you'll find the usual suspects: industrially produced junk food, refined sugar, white flour and cheap, chemically processed fat, together with raw and cold foods and drinks that inhibit digestion.

But you'll also find some traditional products whose inclusion will be surprising to some, such as cheese and other naturally preserved foods. These are foods that have long been recognised as inhibitors of digestion in traditional Asian cultures, and some Western cultures too. Hippocrates, for example, was no fan of cheese, identifying it as a food that could profoundly disagree with certain constitutions. These are views that are increasingly confirmed by modern research.

Junk food

Paracelsus, arguably the father of modern pharmacology, once said, "Too much of anything is poisonous." His words have resonated through the ages and his wisdom should definitely be applied to the modern diet, particularly when it comes to those nutritional *bêtes noires* of the West – salt, refined sugar and cheap fat. These are the mainstays of industrial food, what has come to be called junk food, and they really do need to be avoided.

Why **do** we crave bad food?

Earlier, I talked about how food industrialists pack their products with salt, sugar and fat, for the simple reason that they know that these foods create compulsion. We find these simple, cheap ingredients incredibly hard to resist.

These manufacturers are playing on what was once a human survival mechanism. In the old hunter-gatherer and early agricultural days, human beings developed an obsession with two types of food that are rare, or difficult to find, in nature: calorie-dense foodstuffs like honey and fat, and mineral salts, sodium chloride in particular, which, away from the sea at least, is also uncommon. To this end our behaviour was adapted to a dedicated hunt for sources of these foods, and salt licks (inland concentrations of salt), a trait that is shared with other mammal species. And consequently many animal species can be seen to congregate around salt licks, as well as to brave bee stings to steal honey from wild hives, and to seek out and relish seeds, fresh kills and other calorie-rich delights.

Today we, and other animals, retain these obsessions. At this point, we would do well to recall the experiment on rats referenced earlier in the book. [52] In this experiment, a number of rats were split into two groups, one fed on a natural diet and the other raised on sugar-, fat- and salt-rich junk food. The junk food rats were then subjected to electric shocks as a condition of eating their junk food; they just kept on eating. They would rather be tortured than be denied their dietary fix; and this, above and beyond their calorific needs.

And when the junk food was taken away and a natural diet put in its place, they refused it to the point of *starving to death*. The rats were truly addicted to junk food. An addictive tendency that, in terms of its neurological basis, was seen to mirror the way that we humans can be addicted to heroin.

Since the brain pathways for these addictive patterns are similar in rats and humans, there is no reason to think that humans are any different from these poor rats in their unstinting, compulsive devotion to junk food.

Most food companies seem to know this. And, unfortunately for the human race, not only do we crave these foods but, because of their historical scarcity, they have a disproportionate effect on our metabolisms. Hence we're still geared up to retain and nurture every calorie of sugar or fructose that we can as extra body fat, rather than excrete it or burn it off. This strategy was valuable in the past because

---

52 Johnson PM & Kenny PJ (2010). Dopamine D2 receptors in addiction-like reward dysfunction and compulsive eating in obese rats *Nature Neuroscience* 13: 635-641

our ancestors never knew when they would come across sugary foods again, but these days it means that we gain, and retain, weight as never before.

We have to take care of our diet from the very beginning, because cravings for and addiction to salt, sugar and cheap modified fat are formed in early childhood, probably even in the womb. What's the practical answer to this distressing modern trend? Cook fresh food! Try not to get addicted in the first place.

This principle is as relevant in our schools and workplaces as in our home kitchens. Cooking fresh food to avoid eating junk food is at the heart of this diet. Only then can we protect our digestion and our general physiology.

Case study

Grace, 48, came to the clinic after two months of regular nausea and dizziness. She had been given antiemetic and dizziness medications that hadn't helped, and her confidence was very low. She was also prone to occasional hot flushes, had red spots around her chin and jaw line and was overweight. The symptoms were not linked to anxiety or stress.

The diagnosis was a weak and "hot" stomach needing strengthening and calming: a stomach-friendly diet. Grace cut out all fruit, raw vegetables, sugar, alcohol and very spicy food. She ate three good meals a day so that acidity could not build up in her stomach. I gave her herbal medicine: stomach tonics and bland and aromatic herbs to regulate stomach motility.

It took three months for Grace's symptoms to disappear completely and they stayed away for some time. However, I saw Grace recently as she had experienced more dizziness and had put on weight – her cake cravings had started to get the better of her and she was eating too much sugar again!

Hard-to-digest foods

Hard-to-digest foods include major food groups that can be viewed as traditional, such as *raw and cold food, preserved foods and very rich foods*. They may also be good quality, in that they are well produced, locally, compassionately and in an environmentally sensitive way. But nonetheless, they are difficult to digest. These sorts of foods that can be part of a healthy diet, but they should be eates in small quantities.

Raw and cold foods

Human beings evolved cooking. As a species it's all we've ever known, and so inevitably it is a key principle of this book. We don't have a cow's "fermentation vat" barrel belly; instead, we process our food before we eat it to make life easier for our digestive systems.

As I said, we don't have "fermentation vat" bellies, and nor do we have "warming oven" bellies. As long as human beings have been around, we have eaten warm food; after all, we evolved as a tropical species. Fast-forward to modern times and fridge-freezers, chiller cabinets and drinks dispensers have become mainstream, with the result that cold soda pop, mineral water, salads and ice cream have become everyday items, rather than rare summer treats. These products now typically form a part of nearly everyone's diet in Britain, even in the depths of winter, giving our digestive systems a significant extra hurdle to overcome.

Since we have always eaten warm food, stomach enzymes have evolved to work optimally at body temperature, around 37°C. At this temperature, the complex three dimensional shapes of the enzymes are just right to fit the chemical constituents of the food, like a key in a lock, and break them down. If we then go on to eat and drink cold food and drinks, the shapes of the enzymes distort – they no longer work since they can't easily latch onto the molecules that they are designed to break down. In this very real, chemical way, coldness inhibits digestion and it creates a *de facto* digestive paralysis. A paralysis that can be exaggerated and distinctly uncomfortable because coldness also inhibits *circulation*. It would be deeply unpleasant to have icy-cold water poured down the back of our necks, so why do we do it to our stomachs?

Combinations to counter cold food and drink:

Savoury food
chilli, paprika, cayenne pepper, garlic, horseradish, mustard seed (commonly seen in traditional recipes that are served cold, such as gazpacho, ceviche, cold beef sandwiches and, of course, Bloody Marys)

Sweet food
allspice, cinnamon, clove, dried ginger, fresh ginger, mace, nutmeg

---

These all work well with sweet flavours, making them particularly compatible with iced offenders like sorbet, ice cream and cold winter and summer cocktails. A good chef or foodie will undoubtedly be able to add to this list. To use spices in this way, you might need to make your own ice cream and cocktails, or persuade your chums, local landlord or chef to get involved.

Combinations to counter raw food:

Dare to cook it! Bananas, Britain's most popular fruit, are a good example. Raw, and especially if they are not properly ripe (they should have brown spots on the skin), they are fibrous and starchy and severely obstruct motility, particularly in children. Sautéed with nutmeg and a tiny pinch of dried ginger, they are a delicious and much more digestible child-friendly food. For salads, it is essential to add a spicy dressing to stimulate motility and secretion, hence the convention of adding black pepper and/or mustard to dressings.

Preserved foods

Similarly important is the *chemical* resilience of food; some foods are very resistant to their large molecules being broken down in the gut, which means that motility and absorption are inhibited. Others have artificial or natural preservatives that inhibit the actions of bacteria and fungi in general. These preservatives therefore inhibit our own gut symbionts, whose digestive action is such an essential component of human gut function.

A crude but informative way to test a food's chemical resilience is to mush it up and place it on a shelf, then see how easily the microbes around it settle and grow, breaking down the nutrients to sustain that growth. Those microbes and our gut symbionts use a similar suite of enzymes, and other chemicals and secretions, to break down food, so the length of time it takes a food to go rotten is an approximate indicator of how digestible it might be to us.

To illustrate the point, let's take an incident from my childhood. When I was a youngster at school, we were learning about the different types of microbes to be found in our environment, in particular yeasts and fungi. One of the experiments we did involved leaving out certain foods to see what grew on them. So we got some jam from the school kitchen, left it out on a plate and waited for the mould to grow. And waited. And waited. The mould never grew. The jam that we delicate little things were spooning into our developing guts every day was so packed with preservative that nothing, absolutely nothing, could grow on it. And this can only mean that the same preservatives would have a toxic impact on gut flora.

In the light of the fact that we now know that artificial preservatives are linked to a number of very serious and fatal diseases, due at least in part to their effects on digestive symbionts, this is rather a sobering example. It has turned me into an avid food-product label reader!

As far as our healthy diet is concerned, it is absolutely clear that we shouldn't be keen on artificially preserved foods. But I'd also like to apply this principle to a different group of foods, foods that have been produced in such a way that they are *naturally* preserved. The preservation process, such as smoking, protects these foods against the effects of bacteria and moulds and, at the same time, renders them harder for *us* to break down.

The main foods that fit into this bracket are cheese, cured and smoked meats, and pastry.

Cheese

In a nation of cheese eaters, it's controversial to say that cheese might be harmful to health. Cheese, it seems, is part of what defines our nation. We have cheeses named after counties, bishops, cathedrals and cities. And cheese tastes good too; it's a concentrated food, packed with fat, protein, salt and sugars, exactly what our bodies have evolved to crave.

Yet there's no denying that cheese is difficult to digest. It's a food that is high-fat and therefore rich, but sour accompaniments alone, such as pickle, can't compensate for this, because it has other stubborn constituents that the digestive system struggles with. Casein, a milk protein, and lactose, a milk sugar, both of which are prevalent in cheese, are very hard to break down in the human gut, particularly in the case of adults, many of whom lack the specific enzyme, lactase, that breaks down the milk sugar.

It is this very indigestibility that has made cheese so useful to us in the past. By turning fresh milk into cheese, we create a store of fat and protein that could last for years; bacteria and moulds struggle to digest it too.

Eating cheese might have broad implications for our health. It can obstruct motility, causing bloating and fatigue, potentially further-reaching inflammatory conditions and severe diseases such as bladder cancer.[53]

---

53 Brinkman M *et al* (2011). Consumption of animal products, olive oil and dietary fat and results from the Belgian case-control study on bladder

But what about our bones?

One of the reasons for the popularity of cheese is its calcium content, which is relatively high. Calcium consumption is, as we know, important for the development and maintenance of strong bones, a vital consideration for a nation like Britain that has such high levels of osteoporosis. Cheese and other dairy products are vigorously promoted by the government and industry lobbies for this reason. Dairy products, it seems, should be a cornerstone of our diets.

Isn't it odd that countries with big populations like Japan and China, whose people eat virtually no dairy products at all, have much lower rates of osteoporosis than we do? Similarly, pre-agricultural humans ate no milk or other dairy products after weaning, but because of the high calcium content of the other foods that they ate, their average calcium intake was typically twice that found in Britain today.[54]

The mid-Victorian working class also ate much less dairy produce than you might expect. Butter was expensive, milk was routinely watered down and therefore not trusted, and when it came to cheese, the working class ate a little hard cheese, rather than soft, but strung it out and wasted little.[55] To demonstrate the point, a budget from the 1830s in Dorothy Hartley's *Food in England* shows as much as six times more spent on butter than cheese.

It seems to be a myth then that dairy consumption alone protects us against osteoporosis. In fact, the evidence

---

cancer risk *European Journal of Cancer* 47(3): 436-442

54 Eaton S & Eaton (1999) The Evolutionary Context of Chronic Degenerative Diseases in Stearns SC (Ed), *Evolution in Health and Disease*, Oxford OUP, p253

55 It is interesting to note that, in traditional terms at least, hard cheese is more digestible than soft as it has matured for longer.

to support the notion that dairy consumption contributes to strong bones in either young or old people is minuscule[56, 57]. This dietary myth is simply a triumph of milk marketing.

The Chinese and Japanese owe their strong bones to fruit and vegetables, bony fish, bone stocks, green tea and fermented soy products, facts that have been confirmed by a number of scientific studies.[58, 59, 60, 61] In other words, there are many foods other than dairy products that have high levels of calcium and the other nutrients necessary for strong bones, and these foods are much easier for our bodies to break down and assimilate than cheese.

In my clinic I see a lot of parents who are anxious about their children not getting enough calcium if they give up cheese. The table below is designed to put minds at rest; from a nutritional perspective, there are plenty of calcium-rich alternatives.

56 Lanou A et al (2005). Calcium, dairy products, and bone health in children and young adults: a reevaluation of the evidence, *Pediatrics* 115(3): 736-43

57 See also Dr John Briffa's *Escape the Diet Trap*

58 Yano K et al. (1985). The relationship between diet and bone mineral content of multiple skeletal sites in elderly Japanese-American men and women living in Hawaii. *American Journal of Clinical Nutrition*, Vol 42, 877-888

59 Cooper C et al. (1992) Hip fractures in the elderly: a world-wide projection. *Osteoporos International*, 2: 285–289

60 Muraki S et al. (2007) Diet and lifestyle associated with increased bone mineral density: cross-sectional study of Japanese elderly women at an osteoporosis outpatient clinic. *Journal of Orthopedic Science* 12, Number 4, pp317-20

61 Zhang Y et al. (2007) Calcium intake pattern among Japanese women across five stages of health behavior change. *Journal of Epidemiology* Vol. 17(2): 45-53

Food	Approx. calcium level (mg/100g portion)
Kelp	1200
Hard cheese Sesame seeds	680
Sardines Tofu	510
Almonds Amaranth Figs (dried) Parsley	210-250
Kale (cooked)	180
Black beans Chickpeas Pistachio nuts Quinoa Sunflower seeds Watercress	140-170
Milk Yoghurt	120
Broccoli Cottage cheese Eggs Salmon	40-80

The calcium content attributed to specific foods varies greatly in different sources, and depends on how foods are grown, processed or tested. Tables and charts are also often set out deceptively to favour dairy foods, either by varying portion sizes, or changing the unit of measurement or putting the dairy produce at the top of the list. I have therefore had to use a number of sources to draw up the table above.[62]

---

62 for example National Institutes of Health factsheet, NHS factsheet, McCance & Widdowson's *The Composition of Foods* (see footnote 4) and Scott & Barlow (2002) *Herbs in the Treatment of Children*

Case study

Rory, 12, had been diagnosed asthmatic for eight years. He came to me because he frequently got coughs and colds, with shortness of breath, wheezing and lots of phlegm. The aim was to strengthen his immunity so he got fewer bugs and also to reduce his dependence on medication.

Traditionally speaking, the three main phlegm-forming foods are sugar, white wheat flour and cow's milk dairy products, particularly cheese. Rory was very cooperative in reducing these foods massively in his diet. No more baked potatoes with lashings of Cheddar in the school canteen! I also gave him herbs that are known to help clear phlegm and herbal tonics to strengthen immunity and lung function.

Rory improved steadily over the next few months. He would get coughs but they lasted less time and were less intense. He also had less need for his medication. At the time of writing, he has experienced sustained improvement for a year and hardly ever needs to use his asthma drugs.

Preserved meats and smoked foods

The health-related issues around preserved meats and smoked foods, like ham and bacon, are much easier to understand than the issues around cheese.

Like cheese, these products were developed in pre-refrigeration times as a way of prolonging their shelf life, and, like cheese, they are hard for us to digest. Unlike cheese, these products have not been strongly marketed as essential for health!

They are, in fact, the opposite of healthy. Studies have repeatedly linked the consumption of preserved and smoked foods to a range of cancers, so unequivocally that official agencies recently warned parents not to give their children ham, salami or bacon sandwiches in their lunch boxes.[63]

Is this because they are hard to digest? Possibly, and it is therefore sensible to limit such ingredients in our diets.

Having said that, foods such as preserved chorizo sausage and salami are part of traditional Mediterranean diets which are known to be healthy *overall*, and bacon and ham featured in the mid-Victorian diet. They do appear in this book's recipes. The key is to use them in small quantities to add richness and depth of flavour and *always* to combine them with other ingredients such as lemon juice, cider vinegar and the like so that their richness can disperse in the dish and so that the acids and antioxidants, can start to break them down before we come to eat them.

Above all, when it comes to foods like ham and bacon, *quality matters*. A preservative-free naturally produced product made from very high-quality meat is a much healthier option than a sort of ham-like, died-pink, preservative-packed alternative. Needless to say, most of the ham consumed in Britain is in the latter category, which is why we have been so strongly recommended not to give it to our children today.

---

63 This is consistent with World Cancer Research Fund (WCRF) advice as reported in the *Guardian* newspaper on August 17, 2009

Pastry

Pastry, a combination of fat and wheat flour, is hard to digest by design. It is another food that fails the chemical resilience test; left out, it just sits there for weeks.

In the old days, this property was very useful indeed, because pastry was used as food *packaging*. The famous Melton Mowbray pies, for example, would be put in a chap's pocket as he set out to work in the morning; come lunch time, he'd break off the pastry and tuck into the succulent contents. It was just the same for Cornish pasties. The Cornish tin miners would throw away the dirty pastry having eaten its contents.

So why do we eat so much pastry now? Because it's full of fat and is delicious. But this, combined with the high gluten content of the flour, makes it particularly tough on digestion. I therefore believe that we should eat relatively little pastry as part of a healthy diet. It is so heavy that it bogs us down in our cold and damp climate. When we do eat pastry, as a special treat, of course, it should *always* be combined with digestion-enhancing accompaniments. See below.

Can we make pastry healthier?

A good friend of mine is a pie maker. His recipes are traditional and made with butter pastry; he's committed to making his product as healthy as he can. The mid-Victorians ate pastry in pies too. But mid-Victorian pastry would have been markedly different from that of today. The sort of pastry that the Victorians ate combined thermally stable and nutritious free-range animal fat like butter or suet with old-fashioned wholemeal, low-gluten wheat flour (like today's spelt flour). The modern

---

industrial version is completely different in all its ingredients; it combines high-protein white flour with industrially modified (cancer- and heart-disease-causing) plant oils. The differences are more or less absolute.

Can pastry be healthy? I believe that it can, as long as it remains a relatively small part of overall diet. And only if it is made in a traditional way, with suet or butter and spelt. It remains, however, a rich food, so the strategies for enhancing digestibility outlined below are important.

Combinations for hard-to-digest foods:

Cheese
To counter its stubborn fat cheese needs a sour condiment. To counter its stubborn protein it needs *spice*. This is why a good spicy pickle is traditionally combined with cheese. Ideally, make your own and use lots of vinegar and sour ingredients like green tomatoes, combined with mild aromatic spices like cinnamon and cloves, with something with a bit of punch like a chilli.

Pastry
A similar pickle enhances the digestibility of pastry, composed as it is of stubborn fat (shortening, industrially modified fat, butter, suet or other fat) and stubborn protein (gluten). Another strategy is to

accompany pies and pastries with a spiced fruit jelly or purée (see p. 277 for our spiced damson purée).

Preserved and smoked meats and fish
The crucial flavours for these foods are sour, made more palatable by spice. When preparing smoked mackerel, for example, marinade it in lemon juice first, even if only for a few minutes. The acids in the juice react with the protein and fat of the fish, effectively predigesting it. Then add plenty of black pepper to stimulate gut motility. The same principle is classically applied to smoked salmon.

For bacon or ham, mustard is a typical spicy condiment, combined with the sour of gherkin, sauerkraut or other pickled vegetables. Also, try the tomato ketchup recipe (p. 276). It is an ideal accompaniment to these hard-to-digest foods.

7.

How and Where to Get the Best Food

It is important to include in the narrative part of the book a section on sourcing ingredients. Now that you've got a good idea of what you w*ant to cook, and how to cook it, it is vital to know where and how to get the food.

In this respect, I like to focus on three principles, all of which are key to our building a healthy relationship with food:

- Seasonal
- Local
- Well produced

Eating seasonally

One of the striking aspects of Japanese and Chinese cooking is their continued and passionate use of seasonal ingredients. This a dietary principle was a major contributor to the health of the British nation in the past, and is just as relevant to us today.

Japan's love affair with the seasons can be quite beautiful. In early March, the nation luxuriates under a soft fragrant blanket of plum blossom and the flowers are widely used to decorate favourite soup dishes. As the weeks pass, the famous cherry blossom season begins. As the cherry blossom fades, there is a natural transition to peach blossom. Each type of flower indicates a different stage of spring, heralding the use of special ingredients and recipes.

In the days before the development of refrigeration and the advent of air freight, food *had* to be seasonal. There was no alternative. Inevitably, this dictated the pattern of food shopping and eating: what was available, what had grown well from year to year and what suited purses and household needs.

Fast-forward to the Britain of today, and the picture is quite different. Nearly every food is available year round and cookbooks rarely have significant seasonal content. Therefore we tend to decide what to eat from a recipe, then go out and buy the ingredients, without looking out of the window or referencing a calendar.

This modern habit of ours has an inherent lack of sensitivity that detaches us from our health, climate and environment. It means that we're effectively eating to other countries' seasons and food varieties; in July, when green beans are romping off allotments and garden vines across Britain, the supermarkets are stacked up with air-freighted Kenyan beans. Similarly, we are offered South African apples in July when once early-season British apples would have been eaten. Extraordinary.

The likelihood is that, with the terminal decline of our oil reserves, transport, refrigeration and intensive food production costs will rise to the point where it will make economic sense to re-establish the culinary status quo of the mid-Victorian era in contemporary Britain. Then Britain as a whole will once again eat seasonally. Even if the economic arguments never quite add up, though, we ought to be considering it now, as there are compelling health arguments involved.

There is a wonderful elegance to the match between seasonally available foods and our dietary needs in Britain. In late autumn and winter, starchy root vegetables, nuts and seeds, intense bitter greens (like kale and Brussels sprouts) and fatty meat and fish, together with preserved foods such as pickled, salted and fermented fish, are most available. Which is just what we need, when the climate is persistently cold and damp, warranting rich, sustaining food and strong bitter, spicy and sour flavours to help us digest it.

In late spring, summer and early autumn, lighter greens, fresh beans and soft fruit can be eaten in abundance straight out of the field (with a little cooking of course!), combined with the right mix of refreshing sour flavours and cooling aromatic herbs, or warming aromatic herbs and spices, according to the prevailing weather.

So, despite the current crazy and unnatural abundance of unseasonal imported food, we would do well to eschew it by choice. In the age of the internet, ignorance can no longer be an excuse; there are many good websites with accurate information on seasonal food availability and local providers. There are also plenty of further references to the seasons in this book, in the Short Guide to Herbs, Spices and Medicinal Foods (Chapter 9), the recipe commentaries, and under "Spring", "Summer", "Autumn" and "Winter" in the index.

If we follow this seasonal route, over time our dietary culture will regain its sophistication, particularly in relation to climate and health. An example from Okinawa: the big Okinawa study suggests that the increased consumption of bitter melon (goya) during hot weather is one of the main reasons that the Okinawans outlive their mainland counterparts. Without its moist cooling bitterness, the intense heat of the summer would cause an increased incidence of poor sleep, irritation and inflammation. With its distinctive benefit, harmony is maintained to sustain long life.

It remains for us to create, rediscover and adopt equivalent British strategies. For example, as the chilly wind and rain sweep in from the west with the onset of spring, an ideal way to start the day would be to drink a bowl of chicken broth with fennel, onion and a dash of Worcester sauce. Such a soup has wonderful warming and dispersing aromatic qualities to counter the driving damp and residual coldness of this time of year. The Chinese and Japanese would add ginger to this broth, as its warm spiciness is also an ideal antidote to the spring climate. Equally, we could combine the broth with poached fish or chicken and some noodles or really good bread to make a superb, nourishing, seasonal light lunch or supper.

Locally grown food

The key thing about local, seasonal food is that it is more likely to be fresh, and fresh means nutritious, since, with a few notable exceptions, as soon as food is picked, captured or slaughtered it starts to degrade nutritionally. The actions of sunlight, temperature and chemical processes like the oxidising atmosphere break up certain vital nutrients such as vitamin C and omega 3 oils so that they lose their nutritional benefit.

There is no doubt that the fresher food is, the more likely it is to retain high levels of the delicate nutrients that give our food that health-enhancing "X-factor". Sustained on food that has not lost too much of its natural nutritional goodness, the body becomes much more resilient; immunity is strong, the constitution is protected and we are far better able to deal with our day-to-day challenges.

Time and time again, studies of the world's longest-living populations demonstrate that the fact that they eat so much locally produced, super-fresh food confers significant health benefits[64].

There is an exception to the seasonal, local food rule, and that's for vegetables and fruit that are grown in heated and lit greenhouses hydroponically. This system extends the growing season of foods considerably, meaning that a wide variety of vegetables such as tomatoes and cucumbers can be produced in Britain where previously they might have had to be imported. But I'm not a fan. Instinctively I don't like the energy-intensive nature of such horticulture. I feel it can only be environmentally damaging. Above all, though, it's nutritional issues that are of concern. There is a lack of really good, unbiased research comparing the nutritional value of hydroponic foods with foods grown in a natural way, so there is nothing to dispel my worry that the medium in which these products grow offers only a limited scope in its *range* of nutrients. Microbes, worms, fungi and other small organisms in soil produce chemicals and

---

64 Okinawa is a good example of this benefit

interact with plants in ways which have not yet been explored, so we do not know how they might be of benefit. These vital soil organisms are deliberately kept out of hydroponic systems, meaning that the range of chemical nutrients that hydroponic plants are exposed to is very low indeed. This can only be reflected in the food itself, resulting in a lowered nutritional diversity. On this basis, I suggest that it is best to avoid hydroponically produced foods.

Well-produced/organic food

In nutritional terms, the more food that we can eat that is produced organically or according to an organic/chemical-free style, the better. A number of studies highlighting the enhanced nutrient content of organic over intensively produced foods have already been mentioned in this book. There are plenty more besides, which reinforces the rule of food purchase – buy the best quality that you can afford.

In an ideal world, home-grown food is the best around. It is harvested and immediately eaten – the ultimate guarantee of freshness and quality; a compelling argument for us all to get our names down for an allotment, or to link up with a market gardener.

It is only in modern times, since the advent of petrochemical-boosted agriculture, that the passion for home-grown food has diminished. Food used to be much more expensive and people once made a huge effort to make savings where they could by recycling scraps through keeping pigs and chickens, and growing vegetables and fruit. In early Victorian times, this wasn't just a question of healthy living: it was often a matter of survival. But it created habits that lingered into the next generation. Mid-Victorians often kept a pig and some chickens in their back yards while the rest of their food was organically produced by today's standards.

Today, such practices – despite a rationing-induced revival in the Second World War – are rare. But they can still be found in most societies. In Australia there is an expression, the "Greek Garden", which originally referred to the gardens of Greek immigrants who got the most out of their suburban plots, despite the availability of abundant cheap food in the shops. They planted lemon and other fruit trees, had a veggie patch and always had chickens.

I feel a kindred spirit with those Aussie Greeks. Growing up in Camberwell in central London, feeding the chickens was a wonderful ritual for me too. They ate all our scraps and turned them into eggs, along with plenty of poo for great compost.[65]

The copious supply of free food and the recycling of nutrients that characterise the Greek Garden approach are becoming more and more relevant as food prices rise. They also have other benefits. For example, producing your own food saves a gym subscription as it incorporates a wide range of activity, builds physical fitness and emotional well-being. The same exercise also stimulates gut motility while exposing us to the soil and a well-controlled, relatively pristine environment abundant with symbiotic bacteria. The external ecosystem always sustains the internal one.

---

65 I note that it is now against the law to feed kitchen scraps to chickens. Presumably this is on the basis of hygiene, but I wonder how long such a distinctly modern ruling will last, as foods, especially eggs, get more and more expensive

Case study

Bethan, a 40-year-old female, had been treated for ovarian cancer with chemotherapy, which had induced a premature menopause. She came to me for therapeutic support as she was about to embark on IVF to have a baby using her own pre-frozen eggs. Before seeing me, she still had some monthly bleeding but was told that this was not a period but an illness and was put on a drug regime to stop the bleeding. The monthly bleeding wouldn't stop! I told Bethan that I thought the doctors were wrong and that she still had a menstrual cycle and that she could conceive naturally. Sure enough, after four months of natural treatment, Bethan conceived and went on to give birth to a beautiful healthy baby.

Individual cases cannot be scientifically proven but my belief is that her resilience and retention of fertility in the face of cancer and aggressive, destructive drug treatment were down to her diet. Bethan was and still is the most diligent vegetarian that I have ever met. She took daily supplements of nutrients important for vegetarians like vitamin B12, and every day she ate freshly ground seeds, providing high levels of vital plant fats. She was also a keen allotmenteer; for the better part of ten years the fruit and veg that she had eaten was at the most a few hours old, and she ate loads of it. Her diet was almost perfect for a vegetarian and had been for some time.

That's the secret: plenty of ultra-fresh, local, organic food, like the healthiest people through the ages.

How to get food from abroad

Not all food, however, can be home-grown or local. Many foods that form part of a balanced, intelligently combined and nutritious diet don't grow well in this country. We have no option other than to source them from elsewhere.

For most of my life, I have lived in ethnically diverse urban centres characterised by the ready availability of exotic foods: Afro-Caribbean, Indian, Pakistani, Japanese and, of course, Chinese. I am an absolute glutton for these foodstores, ever fragrant and brimming with produce, in particular for their fresh herbs and bagged and ground spices.

Historically speaking, the trade in these products has made the world go round. Great "spice wars" have been fought over them, including a series of spats between the British and the Dutch. The Silk Route was based on them and it was thanks to the trade in spices that Arab merchants crossed the known world transmitting literature, astrology, mathematics and medicine. We owe a massive debt to these spices for the development of our culture.

It's not just spices that we have obsessively sourced from foreign climes. Other important foreign foodstuffs include grains, like rice and millet, seeds such as quinoa, sesame and sunflower, and nuts like macadamia and cashew.

Many medicinal foods come from abroad. These exotic but remarkably health-enhancing foods have occupied an esteemed place in our dietary culture for hundreds of years, as demonstrated by the writings of Elizabeth Freke, and well-known classics such as Culpepper's *The English Physician*. Medicinal foods were once highly valued in Europe: in the eighteenth century ginseng could cost more than its own weight in gold.

Today, despite transient obsessions with a limited number

of "superfoods", genuine medicinal foods have declined in our consciousness to become far too small a part of our own culture, yet they are undoubtedly crucial elements of a balanced and healthy diet. Hence, the Short Guide to Herbs, Spices and Medicinal Foods (Chapter 9) contains information about walnuts, chestnuts, wolfberry fruit, shiitake mushroom and black sesame – all constitutional tonics greatly valued by traditional dietary cultures, including our own British nutritional cultures of the past. It is no coincidence that walnuts, chestnuts, oysters, curry spices and black pepper were so important to the mid-Victorians; they had an exceptional impact on their health. We now need to recover that lost ground.

How to become an expert

In past ages in Britain, people of all classes had much more *possession* of their food. They knew when it grew, where it grew best, what to eat and what it should cost. Remember how the mid-Victorian working class drank relatively little milk, especially in the cities? It was routinely watered down by unscrupulous merchants – working men and women couldn't get the quality, so they didn't buy it.

Similarly, eighteenth-century Britain was characterised by food price riots or *taxation populaire* – when the goods from a shop were seized by peasants who considered the price of grain unfair. The peasants then simply gave a reasonable price to the merchant, set him free, took the food and went home. More often than not the instigators and perpetrators of these riots were housewives.

Such a passion for and connection with food is no longer a general characteristic of modern Britain. Instead, in the last few decades, we have seen the consumption of ready meals and industrially produced food sky-rocket, to the point where many of us are almost completely disconnected from what we eat. This massive shift in the dietary habits of our society has, as I have explained, large implications for health.

Emulsifiers, trans-fats, flavourings, modified corn starch and the like that tend to be so abundant in factory-produced foods are unequivocally toxic to us. As are the vast quantities of salt and sugar used in these products.

It is easy to see how damaging products like ready-made pizza, oven chips and pre-fabricated curries are for us; they're loaded with the bad guys: chemical additives, modified fat, sugar and salt. But this dietary malaise runs deep; it's subtle stuff and the food corporations' marketing gurus have become masters at pulling the wool over our eyes.

Fromage frais

Let's take an important mass-produced "health food" as an example: fromage frais. Nothing is more minutely scrutinised than the foods that our children eat. Yet this particular "health food" is often marketed specifically for children and it frequently slips through the net.

There is a significant range of fromage frais on the market today. The most popular brands are consumed by the tonne in Britain, and there is no question that broadly speaking we consider them to be healthy. They are promoted as being high in calcium with added vitamins, good for growth and good for bones. Yet we should be suspicious of mass-produced flavoured

---

versions such as strawberry fromage frais.

Fromage frais (literally translated from the French as "fresh cheese") has only one major ingredient in its production – cow's milk; we should buy it as such. If we want to turn it into strawberry fromage frais at home, it's easy. We add... strawberries! A fruit that, if it's not in season, can easily be taken out of the freezer. And if we want to sweeten it up a bit, how about some lovely local honey? You can also add a few aromatic spices such as nutmeg, mace or dried ginger to help cut through the richness of the dairy,

The mass-produced stuff routinely contains added sugar, water, fructose (that's *extra* sugar), colour (unspecified), concentrated juices and extracts, gum stabilisers, modified starches, flavourings (also unspecified!) and acidity regulators. And, believe it or not, that's just in one pot.

This is only one of the items that demonstrate how virtually any industrial food product has a deeply toxic nature, often in direct contrast to the health claims made on the packaging. Further examination of the ingredients reveals why:

- Sugar and refined fructose – ingredients linked to diabetes, obesity, heart attacks and stroke
- Modified maize starch – a cheap thickener of little nutritional value
- Colour, stabilisers, flavourings – typically nutritionally useless
- Processed concentrated juices and extracts, many

of which remain unspecified on the packaging Ironically, the natural version is also very convenient, because fromage frais is a fermented product and keeps well in the fridge; similarly, honey sits on the shelf and most fruit can be stored in the freezer. All in all, then, we can see that natural fromage frais is not only far healthier, but also more cost-effective than the mass-produced flavoured versions.

I am being neither melodramatic nor overly sensational when I say that, like the children who eat these mainstream food products, those of us who regularly eat industrially processed food – and that's most of the population of Britain – are poisoning ourselves, day by day. That's why most of the affluent world is experiencing this extraordinary epidemic of preventable disease.

This means that, at the most, additive-laden factory food should be a rare treat, because, however cleverly it is marketed, it can never be as healthy as fresh, locally sourced, seasonal, well-produced and home-processed food. If we get into the habit of choosing our own ingredients and cooking them at home, not only will our food be fresher and more nutritious, but we will also avoid a bevy of hidden and not-so-hidden industrial additives that do so much damage to our health.

This means that each of us, in our own way, needs to become a food expert. Following the advice in this book is one way to address this need, as it aims to help you rebuild your connection with what you eat, and understand how it is impacted by climate, lifestyle and environment.

Specialist retailers

We should not ignore a very important source of products and information – the specialist retailer. These are the real experts. Many of us are already lucky enough to know that an experienced butcher, fishmonger or stall holder will be able to share valuable advice on the provenance of his goods. Also, he can supply a greater variety of produce such as cheap cuts, bones and offal, which spoils easily – and teach us how to cook it. These cheap foods are some of the most nutritious around, and yet they are often entirely absent in supermarkets, dependent as these businesses are on "just in time" centralised distribution systems.

Bones

Bone stocks are the bedrock of virtually every traditional cuisine in the world, and yet bones and carcasses can be readily obtained only from a good butcher. By choosing to shop at our local butcher and buying these sorts of ingredients we can get cheap, exceptional food, fabulous advice and a chance to build a great friendship with a neighbourhood retailer.

Supermarkets

How do I use supermarkets? As convenience stores, to get cheap fuel and nappies at 9pm on a Saturday, for example. If we all did this, our food heritage would have a chance of returning, rather than forever being on the wane.

A couple of other strategies are worthy of mention:

Bulk purchases

I buy foods like rice, barley, flour, beans, noodles, pasta, honey, maple syrup and tea in bulk from a local wholesaler, cutting costs and reducing the need to go out and buy them all the time.

The internet

For specialist items like dried mushrooms, *gou qi zi* (wolfberry fruit), certain teas and spices, the internet is often the place to turn to, as long as you can establish the reputation of the supplier and end up with a high=quality and good-value product.

Through making these small but vital choices about when and where we shop, we can transcend the modern barriers that are all too often placed between us and our food. Barriers that exist, for example, in the form of cellophane and packaging. And barriers to real understanding of our food, which are erected in other ways, too, such as shipping it in from wherever it is cheapest, regardless of seasonality and quality of production.

THE BE-YOUR-OWN-NUTRITIONIST SHOPPING LIST

Staples	These should be drawn primarily from the table on p. 106. They are chosen for their digestibility and ability to provide sustenance. If you are focused on diet for weight/fat loss then you will need to adapt and expand these lists of foods creatively to include a wider range of fat- and protein-rich alternatives as discussed in the weight loss section p. 180.

Fats and oils	These fall into two categories:
	• Fats for cooking – clarified butter/ghee, dripping or tallow, lard, goose or duck fat, coconut oil
	• Fats for eating – butter, dripping, hemp oil, rapeseed oil, sesame oil, walnut oil, cobnut oil, olive oil
Fermented foods	There are a lot of options here. I typically use soy sauce, Thai fish sauce, black bean sauce, anchovy sauce, Worcester sauce, mushroom ketchup, vinegars (cider, red and white wine, rice), wine, yoghurt, chorizo (fermented sausage), hard cheese and miso, pickles, sauerkraut, real ale, local organic cider
Veg, fruit and mushrooms	These should be seasonal when eaten fresh. When sourced from the wild, market gardens, farmers' markets, home-grown or gifted from allotments they inevitably will be. Some but not all greengrocers use local producers.
	Otherwise seasonal food websites are great sources of inspiration. Here are the locations of useful lists in this book:
	Vegetables – spicy/aromatic p. 90, bitter p. 87, staples p. 106, Short Guide to Herbs, Spices and Medicinal Foods (Chapter 9) p. 198
	Fruit – Short Guide to Herbs, Spices and Medicinal Foods (Chapter 9) p. 202
	Mushrooms – Short Guide to Herbs, Spices and Medicinal Foods (Chapter 9) p. 203

Bread	This needs to be a high-quality artisanal loaf of the sort described on p. 105. Alternatively, you may be into home baking. I don't rate bread machines, though, as the dough never proves for long enough; they rely on large amounts of fast-acting yeast. Getting good bread normally requires a trip to the baker. I rarely see a really good loaf in a supermarket.
Meat, fish and eggs	Meat – see the Short Guide to Herbs, Spices and Medicinal Foods (Chapter 9) p. 204. It is best to focus on cheap cuts and offal, including kidney, liver and tongue. I often buy pork belly, beef shin and good-quality sausages. Bones for stocks come from good butchers. Fish – alas, fishmongers are losing the battle with the supermarkets; a shame, as they provide knowledge and really fresh produce. Aim for variety (and sustainability – we want our children to be able to eat fish too), cook with whole fish (gutted, of course), use the bones for stocks and enjoy UK-sourced shellfish. Eggs – some people have their own chickens, otherwise organic eggs are the most nutritious. It is fun to eat eggs from other birds. Quail eggs, for example, are a revered constitutional tonic.
Beans	See the Short Guide to Herbs, Spices and Medicinal Foods (Chapter 9) p. 201 The best beans are fresh or dried. Recently, I have gone off tinned beans as research suggests that the plastic linings of the tins release chemicals such as BPA which may cause cancer, and other illnesses.

Snacks/Appetisers	Snacks – clients often wonder about snacks, especially for children. It is important not to snack too much or digestion never gets a rest and becomes weak, with consequent illness. There is, however, normally a hole to fill mid-afternoon, or if like me you have a lightning quick metabolism, you will need to eat something every three hours. If I don't, I get ratty! Here are some ideas: Nuts and seeds (like walnuts, chestnuts, pumpkin and sesame seeds), good bread and butter/dripping, dried fruit, soup, pancakes, dried meat or fermented sausage, relish, potted meat, paté, corn on the cob. See also "Street food" in the index. Raw fruit should be limited, local and eaten only in season; raw fruit in the depths of winter is likely to weaken digestion. Chinese snacks are hugely varied and typically highly digestible, although modern versions often contain too much sugar. Examples include steamed buns, lychees, dumplings, noodles, persimmon cakes, smashed-bean buns. Sushi is a brilliant snack if out and about, especially in summer (the cold, raw food element is mitigated by the hot wasabi and the spice of the preserved ginger) Appetisers – you can choose from a wide range of foods, from olives and walnuts to spicy pickles and salted fish. See "Appetisers" in the index.

Condiments	These add vital digestibility value to food, especially rich dishes. In my cupboard/fridge I have brown sauce (good old-fashioned variety), homemade tomato ketchup (p. 276), spiced damson purée (p. 277), curry chutney, real ale chutney, apple and tomato chutney (p. 272), wholegrain mustard, pesto and spiced beetroot pickle. It is best to make mint and horseradish sauces from fresh ingredients as they go off easily.
Tea and other infusions	Green tea is much kinder to digestion than black, but overall tea is a very healthy drink. See pages 84-86. Other infusions of herbs and spices are valuable for digestion. See the Short Guide to Herbs, Spices and Medicinal Foods (Chapter 9) (pages 192–199) for ingredients you might like to use.

Eating out

It is now the norm, in our crazy, busy world, that both adults in a household work, so the modern reality is that most of us *have* to rely on the efforts of others to feed us – in the form of eating out, takeaway or ready meals.

However, eating out and ready meals are nothing new, and they certainly don't have to be unhealthy. The mid-Victorians were famous for their street food and could choose from a long list of extremely nourishing options, including fried fish on toast, baked potatoes, tripe, pea and ham soup, pies, stews, whelks, jellied eels, winkles, prawns, oysters, roasted chestnuts and hazelnuts.

The availability of cheap home-cooked food in the mid-Victorian era was massively raised by the 1830 Beer Act that ruled that for a small one-off payment, anyone was allowed to brew and serve beer in their house. By 1838 there were over 46,000 beer houses, in addition to the more expensive inns, taverns, hotels and public houses. Naturally, where working folk could get beer they could also often get the good food being cooked on the premises.

Similarly, in China and Japan, good hot food can be bought all over the place; in China there is a food stall, booth or cheap restaurant on just about every street. Consequently, the Chinese don't really have picnics like we do. Why would you bother with clammy sandwiches and cold pie when you can so easily get lovely hot and easily digested food?

In Britain today, the beer houses are long gone, most fast-food outlets are purveyors of greasy, super-refined, sugar-laden rubbish and many cafés look to limp salads, a deep-fat fryer and Chorleywood bread for their rather uninspiring menus. Meanwhile, pubs serve "Home Cooked Food" which doesn't necessarily mean that it's cooked at home at all, and restaurants and gastropubs are too expensive for regular eating. Clients that I have educated constantly lament that they know what to eat, but they just can't get it when they're out and about.

Until we can overcome crippling rents and business rates, and absurd European rules and health and safety laws, the fight to increase the availability of healthy food leading to affordable and truly balanced British food – both inside and outside the home – will be a long, frustrating one. But we can start by encouraging our cafés, takeaways and institutions to be inspired, and use bone stocks and cheap cuts, fresh vegetables, herbs and spices, to serve delicious hot, seasonally adjusted food. Let's get them to offer the same simple, nourishing, balanced but high class grub that we can cook at home.

Case study

I treat many babies and children in my clinic with acupuncture and herbal medicine, but there are often cases where dietary changes alone make all the difference. Like Andrew, an 18-month-old boy, who was a bad sleeper with a poor appetite. I got his mum to cut out his night-time milk drink so that his digestion had less work to do at night. Very quickly his sleep settled and immediately he had more appetite for his breakfast in the morning. She also cut out *all* processed food, so that he got no refined sugar or artificial sweeteners, and all his food was cooked from fresh ingredients, using a hand blender to make sauces toddler-friendly.

Stewed fruit was made for snacks and cow's milk replaced with much more digestible unpasteurised goat's milk. He thrived – and was better behaved too!

BE YOUR OWN NUTRITIONIST
SUMMARY

- Eat mostly cooked food
- Serve food and drink warm or hot
- Eat protein and fat from a wide variety of sources. Eat a richer diet as the weather gets colder – more hearty food!
- Ensure, as far as possible, that you eat fresh and well-produced food
- Balance the flavours for climate and circumstance, focusing on bitter, sour and spicy/aromatic
- Eat fermented foods daily
- Severely restrict or, even better, cut out refined sugar (including fructose), artificial sweeteners and refined wheat flour
- Cut out industrially processed foods like margarine and ready meals
- Restrict cheese, pasteurised cow's milk and preserved foods, especially those with chemical preservatives.

8.

How to Lose Weight

The diet described in this book is unquestionably a diet for health. Is it also a diet for weight loss? Demonstrably it is, as the mid-Victorians who ate this kind of diet experienced negligible levels of obesity, as do today's svelte rural Chinese, whose traditional diet is based on similar principles. Indeed, a lack of obesity is a marked feature of all truly traditional diets. The observation of anthropologists throughout the nineteenth and twentieth centuries, as well as dietary visionaries such as Weston Price, was that those who ate according to well-established traditional wisdom and culture developed and maintained a stable fighting weight. The problems started when they adopted the Western Diet.

This pattern is well documented among populations as diverse as the Inuit, the Kikuyu and Maasai of Kenya and the South Pacific islanders. Even vegetarian Hindus in India have been affected in the same way.

When scientists tracked ethnic Japanese who had emigrated to the US after the Second World War, they found that as they started to adopt the typical American diet, and left their traditional habits behind, the incidence of diseases such as breast cancer rocketed. And of course they started to get fat.

Today the same thing is happening in Okinawa, the last bastion of supreme health in the industrialised world. The younger generations are starting to leave behind their traditional ways and to consume fast food, ice cream and soda in ever increasing amounts and they're piling on the pounds.

One of the ironies of the present age is that, despite the well-resourced and ostensibly sincere efforts of our government agencies and the medical community, the British continue to get fatter. Yet the extent of weight-loss literature, scientific or otherwise, is growing by the day. Could it be that the answers to Britain's weight problem already exist and that we're simply ignoring them?

The problem is that the aforementioned government agencies and medical community have failed to recognise the *genuine* causes of fat gain and obesity. Hence the solutions that predominate today, especially in medical circles, simply don't work. As usual, to find a truly effective method we have to examine their methods critically, then sort the wheat from the chaff.

The science of obesity

The cause of obesity is complex and fills whole books in its own right, and for our purposes I don't need to reproduce it here in detail. A simplified version will do. However, there are two excellent recent books on this subject that are worth reading, Dr John Briffa's *Escape the Diet Trap* and Gary Taubes' *Why We Get Fat and What To Do About It*.

Insulin

These two books focus on the role of the hormone insulin in obesity. It is this hormone – more than any other – that instructs fat cells to take in the building blocks of fat from the blood stream, to lay on the fat, and then to retain it. This laying-on and retention of fat is what results in obesity. The pathological effects of insulin are widely accepted in scientific circles.

In this context, it is not controversial to say that the key to weight loss is to reduce consumption of, or cut out, foods that strongly stimulate the release of insulin. Again, it is uncontroversial to say that the food group that does this more than any other is *carbohydrate*, the group that contains sugars and starches. Yet today the prevailing fashion is for "low fat" diets that are high in carbohydrate! A fashion that disregards the fact that dietary fat does not stimulate significant insulin release, yet carbohydrate does.

This bizarre situation has come about for two reasons: firstly, scientists have become fixated on the *"Calories in – Calories out"* principle, which dictates that it's excess calories that we don't manage to burn off with metabolic activity and exercise that get stored as fat.

However, this idea is bunkum for the simple reason that, if we don't eat enough calories, especially in the form of protein and fat, then our metabolisms slow down. We become tired, listless and less active and we burn fewer calories! We also want to eat more because we're permanently hungry as our diet is not satisfying and doesn't fill us up properly. What this means is that, in the real world, people *cannot* maintain calorie-restricted diets; the endless gnawing hunger that accompanies them grinds them down and in the end most people will become locked into a cycle of yo-yo dieting, unsustainable exercise regimes... and obesity.

The second mistaken belief is that fat makes you fat.

This is surely a strange state of affairs when we consider that, because of the actions of insulin, carbohydrate rather than dietary fat is the main food group that is converted into body fat, since it is dietary carbohydrate that stimulates the release of insulin. Remember: this release of insulin caused by the consumption of carbohydrates like sugar is mainstream physiological science.

This peculiar modern muddle is illustrated by the fact that it is only when people develop secondary diabetes that they are advised to stop eating refined sugar. Why should anyone have to attain diabetic status to be told to stop eating sugar? Why aren't we all advised to cut down on sugar to prevent us getting fat, rather than told to eat more salad, lean chicken and low-fat yoghurt?

There is now a clear understanding of how the view of dietary fat as an obesity villain came about. It is based on misleading scientific research conducted by, among others, a dietician called Ancel Keys – the problem being that Ancel Keys was extremely persuasive and charismatic.

Fortunately, however there are those who have countered the bogus science of the likes of Keys, with a sensible weight loss programme that identifies carbohydrate as the primary obesity offender. Our true weight-loss champions include Montignac, Atkins and Dukan, as well as Taubes and Briffa. Despite criticism of their work from many quarters, it seems that these practitioners have been talking sense after all – they have sold many millions of books between them, and for good reason. And yet government policy remains the same, a policy that is based on a "low-fat" philosophy.

Carbohydrates

So who are the key dietary criminals, the worst carbohydrates of all?

The answer to this question is simple, and it lies in Victorian history. For, while the mid-Victorians enjoyed rude health and experienced little obesity, it was a different story for their late-Victorian descendants. This change took place alongside a substantial increase in the availability of two foods: refined sugar and white wheat flour, both of which are carbohydrates.

The decline of the Victorian population as a result of sugar and white flour intake was no freak coincidence. Throughout the world, when traditional populations started to adopt the Western Diet, they invariably began with sugar and white flour, as these are the easiest to transport without spoiling. And previously healthy people quickly became fat, regardless of income or social class.

Once again, I suggest that the British government should be introducing a "sugar tax" to make sugar prohibitively expensive. This move alone would be the single greatest health initiative of the 21st century.

To emphasise the point, it's worth taking another look at British history. Obesity did exist in Britain before the late-Victorian era but it was only found to afflict the wealthy classes, such as the landed gentry and industrialists. That they were fat is evident from the large number of corpulent Regency portraits on view today. The rich sported their double chins and bulging weskits with pride; it was a badge of their class as only affluent people could afford to be fat. Obesity was restricted to the rich due to the high price of white wheat flour and sugar. Indeed, it was said that you could tell how rich a man was by how rotten his teeth were.

They loved the stuff; some would drink from sugar glasses then eat the glass afterwards. And they ate massive puddings and loaf after loaf of smooth, snowy-white bread.

When the price of refined sugar and white flour fell in the late-nineteenth century, all classes were able to dine out on them. Suddenly everyone could be an aristocrat!

Similarly, when sweet rationing ended after the Second World War, the rush to buy sugary foods was so intense that they had to be re-rationed for another four years. There simply wasn't enough sugar to go round.

Once you start eating these foods, it's very hard to stop. But to lose weight and reduce body fat, stop you must.

The solution

The first step in any weight-loss/fat-reduction plan is to:

- cut out refined sugar and white flour *completely*. That means no white bread, sweets, sugary drinks or puddings. And just about no processed food – this includes even apparently healthier items like baked beans. If you look at the labels on these foods you will see that nearly all of them contain sugar.

This is consistent with the strategies dieticians such as Taubes, Briffa, Montignac and Atkins advocate. By doing this alone you are likely to lose weight. However, for those with stubborn predispositions to weight gain another step may be needed, which is to:

- radically reduce or eliminate from your diet all refined grains, starches and sugars, effectively cutting out the broader carbohydrate groups that raise blood insulin levels when ingested. (This means that you will no longer be eating a small number of staple foods that form part of typically healthy traditional diets, such as white rice)

- cut out *all* processed foods to avoid additives such as maize starch and fructose.

Taking these steps, the vast majority of people will lose weight.

A word on fructose

Fructose, found in large amounts in fruit and processed foods, is a sugar that does not raise blood insulin the way that other sugars do. But it is just as big a cause of obesity, since, once consumed, most fructose is metabolised into fat. Much of this fat is deposited in the liver. Fructose also turns off the body's appetite control system, resulting in over-consumption of food in general.

Because fructose levels are high in fruit, you should cut out fruit juice altogether if you are trying to lose weight. Overall, fruit juice, especially from concentrate, tends not to be a healthy drink as it provides a relatively large volume of very acidic liquid, combined with high sugar levels.

Fructose is also added to many processed foods, such as children's yoghurts, and is a major component of corn syrup, a food manufacturers' favourite.

There is a much smaller group of people who will still struggle to lose weight even on this stricter regime. In this case, *most* carbohydrate has to be cut out of the diet, including starchy vegetables like potatoes, whole grains and beans. This means that many of my recommended staples need to be cut out too, such as oats, barley, rye, spelt, carrots, parsnips and pumpkins. Fruit should also be restricted.

While this does not marry with the mid-Victorian diet, which included these foods, it is important to understand that this is a specific strategy applied in cases where fat is particularly difficult to shed, normally as a result of genetic and hormonal predisposition, rather than an approach to general healthy living. Once you have lost fat and have regained a healthy body shape and weight you can experiment with reintroducing healthy starchy staples. It is important to appreciate, though, that if you have a strong tendency to retain fat, you will never be able to eat dietary carbohydrate in the quantities that others seem to manage.

Beyond this, you may be part of the very small group of people whose hormonal predisposition or addictive tendencies causes a stubborn propensity to gain and retain body fat. You will be in a position where, no matter how hard you try, even by folllowing a severely carbohydrate-restricted diet you will struggle to regain a healthy body shape. At this point, if you haven't already sought it, you need professional help and ongoing support from a nutritionist who already appreciates the true causes of and solutions to fat gain and loss. There are a number of strategies such as the use of certain supplements that may help, but they require experienced supervision and guidance to be employed safely.

***

A low-carb diet is inevitably a richer diet as its protein and fat content is higher than usual, which presents issues of digestibility that will now be familiar. The typical consequence of a fat- and protein-rich diet is that motility is affected, which may be why, especially in the early stages, low-carb dieters experience nausea and stomachaches or feel a bit rotten. The answer is to prepare their meals for digestibility. We know from good traditional principles that fat needs to be accompanied by sour and aromatic flavours, vegetables need to be cooked and, while fatty and protein-rich foods are well suited to our cold and damp climate, we need to add a bit of spice and bitterness to assist motility.

A good example of this is the gaucho diet in Argentina. Gauchos, the cowboys of the Pampas, have a diet that consists almost entirely of beef, accompanied by an extremely bitter infusion called *mate*. Without *mate*, which strongly stimulates secretion and motility, their diet would be hard to digest without discomfort. With the *mate* it is sustaining.

Thus applying the principles of flavour and digestibility set out in this book to a low-carb dish makes it tastier, less "heavy" and altogether more appealing.

Artificial sweeteners in a low-carb diet

These chemicals have a highly destructive influence on the gut flora and disrupt hormonal homeostasis; they are not recommended. Some have been linked to obesity, with people who drink artificially sweetened lemonade consuming more calories than those who drink conventional soda.[66]

---

66 Lavin J *et al* (1997). The effect of sucrose and aspartame sweetened drinks on energy intake, hunger and food choice of female, moderately restrained eaters. *International Journal of Obesity*, 21:37-42

Case study – from Jamie Richards' nutrition consultancy

Dave came to see me in November 2011 weighing in at 147 kg (23 stones), with a number of health issues including severe gout and a chronic digestive imbalance. He had problems sleeping and breathing and was on a cocktail of medications to manage his symptoms. Dave had a personal trainer whom he used two to three times a week but he wasn't changing shape or feeling different; in fact he was getting heavier. It was clear Dave was retaining a lot of water as he was puffy and swollen around his face. He was in a lot of discomfort and couldn't see any solutions on the horizon. We talked about where he wanted to be in the near and the long term: he was 46 years old with a young son, so it wasn't difficult to set some goals and get him motivated.

Dave was a typical "Type A" guy. If you told him to train for ten minutes he wanted to carry on for an hour. Everything was a challenge for him and we worked on changing that mindset so he could be more outward-looking. Dave's diet was typical modern fodder: full of wheat, seed oils, fructose, modified dairy and a vast array of chemically enhanced, processed foods. Like many people, he was convinced a lot of these were so called "health foods". He was also a grazer who rarely stopped to consider his food or its impact on him. We made it really simple for him: lots of eggs, quality meats and fish, an abundance of fibrous low-starch vegetables, plenty of olive oil and initially very little fruit. I asked him to fill a regular-sized dinner plate with food, four times a day. His most common complaint about the plan was that he was eating too much, but the fat fell off him. At the time of writing, Dave weighs 105 kg, is off all medications, has complete resolution of his gout and all his digestive issues. He sleeps soundly for seven hours a night and plays football with his son.

SUMMARY

• Carbohydrate restriction is the key, so that food is predominantly from protein and fat sources with non-starchy vegetables

• Remember to use good traditional principles to enhance digestibility of the richer food

• Take it step by step. If one step doesn't work, move onto the next one and see how far you have to go to lose weight:

Step 1: Cut out refined sugar, fructose, refined wheat and processed foods.

Step 2: Cut out all refined grains (like white rice), fruit juice and alcoholic drinks.

Step 3: Cut out most carbohydrates, including potatoes, whole grains and beans. Restrict fruit and starchy vegetables normally considered healthy, like carrots.

Step 4: Seek professional help. You have a strong hormonal or genetic predisposition to weight gain that needs a more detailed diet plan and ongoing assessment.

9.

A Short Guide to Herbs, Spices and Medicinal Foods

This chapter details foods that have strong actions on digestion and health, with an emphasis on herbs and spices. It is by no means exhaustive, and, indeed, it is important that most of the foods are familiar to you so that you enjoy relating to old friends in a new way from the outset.

Each foodstuff is listed along with its flavours, its actions on digestion and its relationship with areas other than digestion, such as the lungs and nervous system. The properties and associations described are mainly based on tradition, though many of them have been backed up by scientific studies. It is impractical for me to reference these studies here, there are simply too many of them.

This section is easy to cross-refer to from the rest of the book, particularly the recipes.

Herbs

The beauty of this herb list is that most of its constituents can be home-grown, here in Britain – many in a window box. When they are picked fresh, they have the maximum level of light aromatic oils and therefore maximum effect, while the leafy elements have a refreshing quality.

For the annual or deciduous herbs, it need not be a problem that they can be used fresh only when in season, as the leaves can be preserved in oil, frozen or dried to be used in cooking all year round.

Basil	Pungent, bitter and slightly sweet, stimulates motility, secretion and flora. Also said to strengthen the lungs.
Bay leaf	Pungent and bitter, stimulates motility and secretion.
Bitter orange peel	As in marmalade. Bitter, slightly sweet and aromatic, stimulates appetite, motility and gut flora. Used in stocks, soups and stews.
Caper (berry or bud – pickled)	Mildly pungent. Traditionally used in the Mediterranean for healthy joints: the pungency cuts through the obstructiveness of damp. Classically combined with rich meats, sauces and cured fish.
Chamomile	Slightly bitter and sweet, soothes digestion.
Chervil	Bitter and slightly sweet, used to balance strong spices.
Chives	Pungent and slightly bitter, stimulates motility and secretion.
Coriander leaf	Bitter and aromatic, stimulates motility and secretion. Refreshing and balances strong spices.
Dandelion leaf	Bitter, counters hot weather and very spicy food. A noted diuretic, it can help with fluid retention. All parts of the dandelion plant have a culinary use. The flowers can be eaten and the root taken as an infusion.
Dill leaf	Aromatic and slightly bitter, stimulates appetite.

Lavender flower	Aromatic and slightly sweet. The French cook with lavender. Famously calming, it soothes the gut to clear wind and gently strengthens digestion.
Liquorice	Very sweet and slightly bitter, strengthens digestion overall.
Lovage	Bitter and aromatic, stimulates motility and secretion, good in stews.
Marjoram	Bitter and aromatic, astringent (can settle an overactive bowel) and calming for digestion overall.
Mint	Aromatic. Like coriander leaf, this is one of the refreshing aromatic herbs, so it is good in summer, or in combination with very spicy foods or lamb.
Nasturtium (leaves, flowers and seeds)	Bitter, pungent and sweet. The flowers and leaves are broadly equivalent, with bitter and pungent flavours stimulating motility – particularly good for rich foods eaten on a hot day i.e. barbecues! Nasturtium seeds can be pickled and are equivalent to capers.
Oregano	Slightly aromatic and bitter, stimulates motility. Classically combined with cheese or pork sausage.
Parsley leaves and seeds	Slightly aromatic and bitter, stimulates secretion and motility and is a mild diuretic.
Peppermint	Aromatic and slightly sweet. Cools excess spice and soothes the gut. Relieves nausea. Also said to strengthen the lungs.
Rose and rosewater	Sweet, aromatic and slightly bitter. Calms and soothes the gut, stimulating motility, especially where there's emotional stress involved or we're feeling liverish.
Rosemary	Bitter and aromatic, stimulates motility – renowned for treatment of trapped wind. Said to calm the effects of emotional stress on the gut.
Saffron	Sweet, bitter and aromatic, regulates digestion overall.

Sage	Bitter and aromatic, warms and moves the gut to counter rich foods. It is said to soothe the gut and promote healing.
Savory	Aromatic, bitter and slightly sweet, stimulates motility and secretion and is said to strengthen the lungs. Winter savory is traditionally combined with Jerusalem artichokes to mitigate their flatulence-inducing properties!
Sorrel	Sour, a mild diuretic, counters hot weather and very spicy foods.
Sweet Cicely	Aromatic and slightly sweet. Calms the stomach. The leaves and seeds have an aniseedy flavour that mellows sour flavours, so a good summer herb. The aromatic components also combine well with rich ingredients like eggs.
Tarragon	Bitter and slightly aromatic, stimulates motility and secretion.
Thyme	Bitter and aromatic, stimulates motility to counter sluggish digestion, especially in combination with fatty foods. Traditionally said to dry out mucousy lungs.

Spices

Spices are mostly exotic; they don't grow in Britain. They have, however, been part of British cooking for as long as the spice traders have existed, for thousands of years. Many of these will already be familiar to you, but their pivotal role in promoting digestion might not be.

Could be time to restock the spice cupboard!

Allspice (pimento/ Jamaica pepper)	Aromatic. A gentle digestive stimulant said to ease flatulence and stomachache.
Aniseed	Aromatic and sweet, stimulates motility and gut flora. Soothes the gut to relieve flatulence.
Caraway seed	Aromatic and sweet, warms and stimulates motility and gut flora. It stimulates appetite and is said to treat diarrhoea and trapped wind.
Cardamom	Aromatic. Stimulates appetite and motility. Traditionally used to counteract nausea, muggy headaches and gut pain.
Cayenne pepper (red pepper)	Very spicy. A form of chilli pepper that is often ground into a powder. Often added to sauces and condiment recipes and balanced with sour cooling flavours.
Chilli pepper	Very spicy, stimulates motility but needs balancing with other refreshing and cooling herbs and foods.
Cinnamon bark	Strongly aromatic and spicy too, stimulates appetite. A traditional cold and diarrhoea remedy as it is slightly astringent.
Cinnamon twig	Aromatic and bitter, regulates digestion overall and stimulates the lungs.
Clove	Pungent, warms the digestion to specifically counter the stagnation of damp and coldness. Stimulates appetite and regulates intestinal motility to relieve nausea and trapped wind.
Coriander seed	Aromatic. Regulates motility to relieve trapped wind and diarrhoea, especially in children.
Cumin	Aromatic and sweet, warms digestion and stimulates motility and symbionts.
Dill seeds	Aromatic. Traditionally this is the herb of choice for colic in children as it gently regulates motility.

Fennel seed	Aromatic and sweet, stimulates motility and warms digestion. Promotes appetite and relieves spasm, as in trapped wind. Considered a very important mild spice for regulating motility in babies and children.
Fenugreek seed	Very bitter, aromatic, warms digestion. Used to alleviate lower-abdominal pain.
Galangal root	Spicy, more or less equivalent to fresh ginger.
Garlic	Spicy and aromatic, strongly stimulates motility and is said to strengthen the lungs. Proven to promote symbiotic bacteria while killing pathogenic bacteria.
Ginger (fresh root)	Spicy and slightly sweet, regulates stomach motility and secretion, hence its role in soothing nausea.
Ginger (dried)	Strongly spicy. Warms and stimulates motility.
Horseradish	Strongly spicy. Strongly stimulates motility, hence its combination with rich meats such as beef.
Juniper berry	Slightly aromatic and bitter, stimulates motility to aid digestion of rich food. A great way to introduce tasty bitterness to a dish. Try adding it to stews and casseroles.
Mace	Aromatic and slightly sweet, warms and stimulates motility. Regulates symbionts to keep out the bad guys!
Mustard seeds	Spicy and aromatic, warms digestion and stimulates motility.
Nutmeg	Aromatic, warms and stimulates motility. Regulates symbionts just like mace.
Paprika	Bitter, aromatic and slightly sweet, stimulates secretion and motility.
Pepper, black and white	Very spicy, counters stagnation caused by cold and damp.

Star anise	Sweet and aromatic, promotes motility and gut symbionts. A mild spice to combine with puddings and rich meat like pork and beef.
Turmeric	Bitter and pungent, stimulates motility and secretion. Used for reducing pain from trapped wind and bloating.
Vanilla	Sweet, a gentle flavouring that strengthens symbionts and stimulates secretion.

Medicinal Vegetables

Super-fresh vegetables are one of the touchstones of healthy eating, and the more that we grow and cook straight from the plant pot or veg patch, the better. Packed with nutrients, they provide vital nutrition for the metabolism and substance of our bodies.

Beyond the staples, some of the vegetables described below have particularly interesting actions in terms of health and our climate.

Celery stalk	Slightly salty and bitter, balances very hot dry weather. Also ideal to balance the warming and drying nature of strongly aromatic spices.
Chard	Bitter and sweet, traditionally said to soothe the lungs and cool excessive spice.
Chicory/Endive	Bitter and sweet, a wonderful summer vegetable for hot dry weather.
Cress	Aromatic, an ideal summer food that also balances strong spices.
Fennel bulb	Sweet and aromatic, soothes digestion and stimulates motility.

Leek	Aromatic and sweet, stimulates motility and counters the stagnating effect of cold damp climate.
Nettle	Sweet and bitter. This should be viewed as a fresh vegetable, especially in spring when the tips are tender. Rich in nutrients, it is viewed as a blood tonic, while the bitterness means that traditionally it is used as a mild diuretic to regulate the urinary system.
Onion	Aromatic and sweet, stimulates motility and is said to strengthen the lungs.
Radish	Strongly aromatic, stimulates the stomach and is said to strengthen the lungs.
Rocket	Aromatic and bitter, stimulates appetite and motility, a great green leaf for year-round consumption – grow your own!
Seaweed	Salty/savoury and mineral-rich, seaweed is considered one of the key foods responsible for the health and longevity of the Japanese. Intensive farming depletes the mineral content of our soils and hence our foods; seaweed is a good alternative source of them. There are many types of seaweed and Britain has a number of the edible varieties. Be careful if you have a thyroid problem as they are high in iodine.
Spring onion	Aromatic, stimulates the stomach and the lungs, one of the great Eastern culinary vegetables.
Watercress	Aromatic and slightly bitter, stimulates motility and secretion. This is one of the iconic pungent British greens and it is very nutritious.

Medicinal grains

The grains listed below are major British staples, chosen for the valuable role they play in our digestive health. Baked, sprouted, fermented and boiled, they deserve a much higher status on our plates than the ever-present wheat.

Barley	This sweet grain is particularly good for stomach health. It is cooling, calming and moistening and stimulates motility while nourishing symbionts. Also good consumed as barley water. Barley couscous is available.
Buckwheat	Calms the stomach and stimulates motility. Sweet in flavour, it nourishes symbionts.
Millet	Sweet and bitter, stimulates motility and nourishes symbionts.
Oats	Sweet, nourishes symbionts. It strengthens the nervous system, so it is calming in regular small quantities.
Rice	Sweet, a most digestible grain. It is likely that white rice is healthier than wholegrain as it contains much lower levels of compounds like phytic acid that affect iron absorption. Rice has starches that break down at just the right rate to nourish digestion and be healthily absorbed – no wonder it underpins the diet of the most healthy people on earth.
Rye	Bitter, encourages motility and, as a mild diuretic, the excretion of excess body fluids.
Spelt	An ancient form of wheat, brought to Britain by the Romans. It contains much lower levels of gluten than modern varieties and a better nutritional profile. This makes it much more digestible than the modern stuff. People who tend to suffer bloating and significant gut pain after eating normal wheat bread often find that they can tolerate spelt bread. Spelt pasta is also available.

Wheat bran   Sweet, mellow and strengthening for digestion.

Medicinal beans

Beans are splendid food. Many of them have particular medicinal properties that make them especially useful in strengthening and maintaining our health, and countering the effects of our climate.

We live in unusual times. The use of agrochemicals, and the destruction of the rainforests to produce animal feed mean that, overall, far too much low-quality meat is eaten in the Western world. How did we boost the protein content of our diets before this strange state of affairs? Beans!

And, when beans are grown in a responsible way, they enhance the quality of the soil for other vegetables.

Aduki bean	Both sweet and sour, strengthens digestion and soothes the stomach so it protects against the effects of excess spice.
Black bean	Sweet and mild, strengthens digestion and the constitution.
Broad bean	Sweet and mild, stimulates motility and nourishes gut flora.
Cocoa	Bitter and sweet, stimulates motility and secretion.
Green bean	Sweet and mild, strengthens digestion.
Soybean, black (fermented)	Sweet, strengthens digestion and the constitution.
White bean	Sweet and mild, strengthens digestion.

Medicinal fruit

Fruits often have strong flavours and therefore strong effects on digestion and the rest of our health. As part of the government's "five-a-day" campaign, they have been very much touted as a big part of the dietary solution to today's diet-induced health crisis; especially now that they are available year round, rather than just seasonally, due to air freight and rapid sea transport. However, excessive consumption of fruit, especially raw fruit, with its stubborn cell walls and structures, and strong, acidic sour flavours, depletes digestive strength. Fruit can take a lot of digesting!

The best way to deal with fruit, therefore, is to cook it, or combine it intelligently to enhance the digestibility of other foods. Don't eat too much of it, and consume sugary tropical fruit like mangos, pineapples and bananas only as a rare treat.

Crab apple (and other sour apple varieties)	Sour and sweet. Stimulates secretion, particularly to help in digestion of rich meats such as pork or goose.
Elderberry	Bitter and sweet, soothes and regulates the intestine.
Goji berries (wolfberry/ gou qi zi	Sweet and rich, a constitutional tonic. Add to soups, stews, stocks and casseroles and combine with light aromatic spices.
Hawthorn berry	Sour and sweet. Is used in China to relieve indigestion, particularly from eating too much meat and greasy food.
Lemon zest	Bitter and aromatic, balances the effect of very spicy food and stimulates secretion.
Lychee	Sweet and sour, strengthens symbionts.
Pear	Sweet and cooling. Steamed with cloves it is said to clear phlegm from the lungs.

Persimmon	Bitter and astringent, regulates the stomach. Renowned for its use as a relief for belching and hiccough.
Rosehip	Sour and slightly sweet. Stimulates the gall bladder to cut through fat and gently stimulates motility.

Medicinal Mushrooms

Many types of mushroom are used in traditional cooking including the chestnut, button, field and boletus varieties. Others, such as shiitake, maitake and oyster mushrooms are renowned as dietary medicines.

Mushrooms have a strengthening effect on the body, both for digestion and the general constitution. Indeed their medicinal benefits are unique, probably because they are primary decomposers, extracting and creating nutrients that can't be found in other types of organism.

For this reason, and because of their rich and delightful flavours, they are revered in traditional cuisines the world over – the Chinese and Japanese consume more than five times as many mushrooms per head as the Americans! We should work to recreate a mushroom culture in Britain.

Boletus edulis (porcini/ceps)	Sweet, regulates the immune system and nourishes symbionts.
Button/ chestnut	Sweet, stimulates the appetite and nourishes digestion.
Oyster	Sweet, a strong immune tonic.
Portobello	Sweet and savoury, a strong blood tonic.
Shiitake	Sweet, an important blood and constitutional tonic. One of the most popular mushrooms in the world and revered by the Chinese and Japanese.

Medicinal meat, fish and eggs

In this guide, when it comes to meat, offal is king. It has a much higher micronutrient density than the skeletal muscle that obsesses modern British society. It's the favoured meat of just about every traditional society from China, and the Maasai to the Inuit and beyond.

As well as offal, a number of meats, such as chicken and a range of fish have already been talked about in the book as nourishing staples and health-enhancing foods. A few more are worthy of mention since they have a particularly beneficial effect on digestion, blood and the constitution. These are listed below.

Eggs are also included in this list. They are extremely nourishing and should be eaten regularly as part of a balanced diet, as long you have no specific egg intolerances.

When sourcing meat, fish and eggs, quality is very important. If animals have been well looked after, allowed to roam and given access to a varied diet, the meat will have fewer toxic contaminants and a much healthier range of nutrients. This is a crucial dietary principle: healthy animals mean healthy humans.

Carp	Sweet and nourishing. A strong tonic for blood and digestion.
Chicken	Sweet, nourishes symbionts. There was a time when chicken was a rare treat; now it is commonplace but that doesn't stop a really good organic bird being truly medicinal. It is so nourishing and easy to digest.
Eggs	Chicken and duck eggs are sweet, rich and strengthening. Quail eggs are a revered constitutional tonic.

Herring	Sweet and rich. Although an oily fish, it is light enough to be easily digested and a digestive tonic. Also traditionally said to benefit the lungs.
Mackerel	Sweet and rich. An important tonic for digestion and blood.
Mussels	Salty. A constitutional tonic, said to be good for fertility and longevity.
Offal	Includes brains, heart, sweetbreads, liver, kidneys and pluck (lungs and intestines of sheep) Traditionally speaking, the organs are said to nourish the corresponding organ in the human body; chicken liver strengthens the human liver, for example. The logic is compelling as the nutrients more or less exactly match.
Oysters	Salty and sweet. Nourish vitality, blood and the constitution. Said to be good for fertility and longevity.
Quail	Sweet, nourishes symbionts.
Rabbit (wild)	Sweet, nourishes symbionts. Up until the 1950s, more rabbit was eaten in Britain than chicken; it was a very important food! Our diet has changed due to intensive farming methods, which have made chicken more widely available. However, the birds are often stressed and diseased and produce poor-quality meat. Meanwhile, many rabbits have been killed off by myxomatosis. Wild rabbits still have to be controlled, however, so they might as well end up on our plates.
Sardines	Sweet and rich. An important tonic for digestion and blood.

Medicinal nuts and seeds

These provide a number of particularly important nutrients, most notably their essential oils.

In Britain seeds and nuts tend to be served up in bags, salted and roasted, so much of their nutritional value is lost. Elsewhere, the tradition in different. One of my most treasured memories is of watching elderly men and women in a huge tea garden in Sichuan, China. They spent all afternoon eating sunflower seeds and playing cards, the pile of seed husks growing into a little mountain as the time went by. Sadly, these rituals are being eroded in modern China as they have been here in Britain.

Such a cultural loss is also a nutritional loss. The process of cracking nuts and seeds from their shells or husks and eating them fresh, enables us to extract the maximum number of nutrients, and provides a relaxing ritual of preparation to enhance digestive efficiency.

Almond	Sweet and slightly bitter, it is said to strengthen the lungs.
Chestnut	Sweet, a digestive and constitutional tonic.
Flax seeds	Rich and oily. A vegetable source of omega 3 oils, it improves motility in the large intestine to relieve constipation.
Hazelnut	Sweet and rich, can strengthen gut symbionts.
Hemp seeds	Sweet, they moisten, soothe and nourish the gut. Hemp oil is a wonderful locally produced tonic.
Sesame, black	Sweet and rich, a constitutional tonic.
Walnut	Sweet, bitter and rich, a constitutional tonic and ideal winter food.

Medicinal oils and fats

Fats can come from plant and animal sources. Plant oils, fresh, cold-pressed and produced without chemicals, are precious foods. Organic production is particularly important for plant oils because many pesticides are fat-soluble. Not all of these oils are suitable for frying, because high temperatures can alter their chemical structures and reduce their health benefits. But boiling is fine, so they can be used in soups, stews and casseroles, as well as dressings, mayonnaise and dips.

Animal fats are just as valuable. It is notable that our modern fear of animal fats is unfounded and no good for health. When animal fats come from free-ranging, wild or well-husbanded beasts, they do not deserve their bad press. They contain a wide range of essential nutrients including omega 3 essential fatty acids and vitamins. Similarly, in eggs, butter and clarified butter or ghee, animal fats provide vital nutrients for vegetarians. Animal fats are also very important for cooking as they are partly saturated and therefore stable at high temperatures.

Plant fats, by contrast, tend to distort when they get hot, forming cancer- and heart-disease-causing trans fats and other pathogenic chemicals. We already know that the mid-Victorians ate a lot of animal fat and predominantly cooked with saturated animal fat such as butter, lard or dripping. Hence, they had very low intakes of trans fats and associated low levels of cancer, obesity and heart disease.

Today, fried pork fat continues to be a delicacy in parts of China, just as it once was in Britain. Indeed, we still eat pork scratchings today. The expression to "chew the fat" comes from a landlord showing favour to a customer by giving him or her some fat cut from the ham that was traditionally kept behind the bar. It's once more time to give fats the status that they deserve.

Butter	Sweet and rich, a strong tonic for the blood, membranes and nervous system.
Clarified butter/ghee	This is effectively cooked butter. The cooking process removes the milk solids and water, making it more stable at high temperatures and less likely to burn – it is ideal for frying. Sweet and rich, it nourishes nerves and membranes and is relatively easy to digest.
Coconut oil	Sweet and rich. This is a saturated plant fat but one that we should love rather than fear! A tonic for the blood and nervous system. The molecules are small and easy to digest. It is also great to cook with, as its molecules are stable at high temperatures.
Beef dripping/ suet	Delicious and rich. Mid-Victorian standards.
Flax oil	Sweet and moistening, an omega 3-rich oil that soothes the gut. Traditionally used in the treatment of constipation.
Goose fat/ Duck fat	Sweet and moistening. These two fats deserve a mention because they are lighter than most other animal fats because they contain high levels of mono-unsaturated fats, just like olive oil, making them easier to digest. It is thought that goose fat is one of the health-enhancing factors in the French Paradox. Now, of course, we know that the only relevant dietary paradox is that good quality fat is thought of as unhealthy in the first place! If you cook a goose or a duck, *don't throw the fat away.* Cook with it.
Hemp oil	Sweet and rich, this is one of the most digestible oils. Now widely available, it has a fabulous balance of essential fatty acids and is a revered traditional ingredient. This oil is not stable at high temperatures and so is not a good frying oil.

Olive oil (fresh extra virgin)	Sweet and moistening, nourishes all of the body's membranes. The fresher this oil is, the easier it is to digest as it contains some wonderful light aromatic components. The proven health benefits of olive oil are legion, and it deserves its place in the British kitchen.
Rape seed oil	Sweet and rich, this oil is packed with omega 3 fats and is a great dietary option. Go for the good stuff, though, fresh, cold-pressed and well-produced as there are all sorts of problems with "Canola" which is produced with high chemical inputs.
Sesame oil	Sweet and moistening, this oil is an all-round good performer. In particular it enhances the fluidity and flexibility of membranes, resulting in skin nourishment and cardiovascular benefits. Sesame can be used for cooking as it tends to form less nasties at higher temperatures than other polyunsaturated oils.

Medicinal condiments

Some recipes for digestion-promoting sauces and the like can be found later in the book (see "Add-ons"). However, there are a number of simple products and foods that are worthy of consideration in addition to these. Each has a role to play in stimulating appetite and enhancing digestion. Each dietary tradition has its own particular foodstuffs, and the following are just a few of them. The list, otherwise, would be endless.

Cider vinegar	Sour and slightly pungent, refreshes and stimulates appetite.
Miso	Salty/savoury and slightly sour, strengthens digestion in small amounts.
Soy sauce	Sweet and salty/savoury, stimulates appetite and regulates the stomach to reduce nausea.
Yeast (natural, *not* fast acting)	Sour, sweet and bitter, stimulates secretion, motility and gut symbionts. Consume in small amounts to avoid candida.

Others that are worthy of mention are Thai fish sauce, mushroom ketchup, Worcester sauce, anchovy paste or sauce and black bean sauce; they are all salty/savoury and contain fermented ingredients. Therefore, they are highly nutritious and stimulate the appetite.

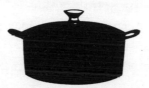

RECIPES

In certain respects we are very lucky to live in the modern age. There is an incredible amount of food information available on the internet, with recipes leading the way on TV channel sites supporting cookery and food shows; celebrity chefs', weight-loss gurus' and food historians' own content-rich sites; blogs and messageboards that provide updates and feedback, improvements and variations on the recipes.

There are thousands and thousands of recipes and reams of food-related comment easily accessible online.

In this context this recipe section's role is illustrative rather than extensive. The small number of recipes presented here aim to show the way, as it were, and encourage you to create your own, based on the same principles. My recipes detail the inner mechanics of the dish, particularly in relation to flavour. Each recipe also has a "variations" paragraph outlining how it might be modified for different climates, seasons, constitutions and proclivities.

I also have more recipes with their own commentaries on my website (www.george-cooper.co.uk), aimed at helping anyone who wants to develop a varied and clearly defined approach to healthy cooking.

Please note that the portion sizes are based on hearty appetites, so you may need to adjust accordingly.

Case study

Dinah, 30, had experienced pre-menstrual stress (PMS) for three years. She could be irritable for as much as three weeks in each 28-day menstrual cycle. When the period came it could be very painful. She also suffered from typical IBS symptoms, rumbling gut, stress-related bloating and variable appetite.

From a dietary perspective, her two main problems were that she didn't eat enough rich food and she didn't eat often enough. I got Dinah eating at least every three hours, and much more meat and fat, employing simple principles to aid digestibility. Using these principles was very important in her case as she was changing her diet signfiicantly, and she was eating more food overall. To generate and maintain interest and variety, Dinah looked up lots of traditional recipes and adapted them for climate, as well as improving their health benefits by substituting with digestion-friendly ingredients and applying flavour principles. She also started taking aromatic herbs for motility, and blood and digestive tonics and herbs for blood circulation.

Very quickly, she felt better, as she had a steady flow of sustenance to her brain and heart. She also gained in strength. Her mood improved and stabilised, the bloating and rumbling in her gut reduced and her period pain diminished.

Simple Recipes

Baked fish with herbs

Serves 2-4

Ingredients

a whole fish, head on, scaled and gutted (mackerel,
bream, mullet, bass, gurnard or pollock)
a knob of butter and 2 tbsp olive oil
1 large fennel bulb, sliced
½ white onion, diced
2cm fresh root ginger, finely sliced
a generous handful of chopped fresh coriander
1 large mild chilli deseeded and finely chopped
½ cup dry white wine
3 slices lemon
generous pinch of salt
½ tsp black pepper

Method

Sauté the fennel, onion, ginger and chilli in the olive oil and
butter for 5 minutes, just to soften them a bit.

Put all the ingredients in a foil-covered dish and place
in an oven at 170°C for 10 to 20 minutes until the fish is
moist and just cooked; cooking time will depend on the size
and type of the fish. Serve with rice, soy sauce and lightly
sautéed fresh veg.

This is a quick, convenient and common way to cook fish
and produces a marvellously light, refreshing result that is

ideal for the British summer.

The refreshing coolness of the dish comes from the sourness of the wine and lemon and the cool aromatics of the fresh coriander, while the lemon pith provides a little bitter undertone which also stimulates motility and refreshes the palate in hot weather.

As a rule, sour constricting astringency from the lemon and wine needs to be balanced with expansive spice to stimulate motility and give warm satisfaction, a task achieved by ginger, chilli and black pepper in this case. Onion and fennel round out the flavours in the recipe by providing sweet aromatics to stimulate appetite and nourish digestion.

This can be a cheap recipe to put together, using less popular whole fish varieties. The use of whole fish instead of fillets adds a little richness and depth of flavour to this dish as the nutrients from the head and bones infuse the sauce.

Variations

A simple version of this recipe involves fish fillets and the other ingredients sealed in a foil parcel and thrown on top of a barbecue. This is ideal for those who find barbecued food rich and cloying – definitely a healthy alternative!

Otherwise, the dish can be made more complex by precooking wine or stock with butter, a small diced onion, a teaspoon of black peppercorns and a heaped teaspoon of juniper berries for 15 minutes. The resulting sauce is then poured hot over the fresh whole fish in a hot pan, which is cooked in the oven for 5 to 10 minutes. The advantage of this more complex method is that it gives the bitter aromatics and spice of the juniper and black pepper time to infuse the sauce. This creates more depth and potency of flavour for enhanced digestion and satisfaction.

Chestnut soup

Serves about 6

Ingredients

50 g butter
3 shallots, finely chopped
2 celery stalks, finely chopped
1-2 cooking apples, peeled and roughly chopped
2 tins chestnut purée (widely available)
1 litre vegetable stock
1 tsp sugar
½ tsp mace
salt and pepper
45 ml medium dry sherry

Method

Melt the butter and fry the shallots for 5 minutes. Add the celery and apple. Cover the pan and sweat the vegetables over a gentle steam for 10 minutes.

Add the chestnuts and pour in the stock, mace, sugar, salt and pepper. Bring to a gentle boil, then cover pan and cook for 30 minutes. Liquidise. Gently rewarm and add the sherry just before serving.

This recipe doubles as a winter delight and a particularly nourishing dish for vegetarians. And it is beautifully balanced, with representatives of all the flavours, bitter (celery), salt, sweet (chestnuts and sugar), sour (apples) and aromatic/spicy (sherry/mace/black pepper).

The nourishing quality of the dish comes from the chestnuts, which are a famous sweet digestive and constitutional tonic. The addition of a small amount of sugar enhances the tonic sweetness of the chestnuts.

Variations

There is nothing to say that fresh chestnuts can't be used for this recipe; it's a bit fiddly, but the result is absolutely delicious. Steam them, peel them, then whiz them up with a bit of stock to make the purée.

You can also adapt the recipe in particularly perishing weather by adding more aromatic spices to counter penetrating cold and damp. Cinnamon, nutmeg and a little dried ginger are perfectly suitable.

Chicken noodle broth

There are no amounts or exact instructions here, although there are some ingredient-specific suggestions in brackets – mirrored in the "method" text. The key with this recipe is to embrace the concept and then play around with variations. In this recipe we have the goodness of the whole chicken, combined with a host of beneficial ingredients and flavours that stimulate the senses and digestion.

Ingredients

whole organic chicken
1 chopped onion
a handful of chopped celery
lemon grass (2 sticks)
ginger (2 tsp)
garlic (2 cloves)
fresh turmeric (2cm fresh root or 1 tsp powdered)
live miso (1 tbsp)
limes (2)
lime leaves (6)
pak choi (4 heads)
spring onions (4)
thick noodles
soy sauce (1 tbsp)
coriander (a handful)
sweet basil (a handful)
mushrooms of some kind (200 g)

Method

Place a whole organic chicken in a large pot and cover with

water. Add chopped onion and celery. Bring to the boil, skim and then simmer for around an hour.

Remove the chicken and leave it to cool while you strain the stock and return it to the pan. If you have more stock than you need, put half of it to one side for the moment. To the other half add two or three crushed lemon grass stalks (use the base of a saucepan or a rolling pin) and then a large thumb-sized piece of ginger, some fresh turmeric and two or three cloves of garlic, all finely chopped or minced. Add about six kaffir lime leaves and a tablespoon of light miso. Keep the broth simmering while you begin to strip the meat off the chicken. Add as much of the meat as you like and reserve the rest for another meal or two. Now add some noodles. It pays to have good-quality noodles as they soften nicely in the soup.

Add some greens like pak choi, chopped spring onions, a good splash of soy sauce and plenty of lime juice. Right at the end add two handfuls of chopped coriander and some sweet basil. Lastly, you can break up the chicken carcass and return to the leftover stock. Add some more water and add a good dash of white wine vinegar to help release the goodness from the bones. Add some more onion and celery and simmer it for another two hours at least. Strain it off and allow it to cool. It will refrigerate well for three days or freeze for longer.

In some ways this dish is very similar to classic Thai fish curry. The bones as well as the meat of the animal are used to create a nutritious sauce, while spices are used to stimulate motility and secretion to efficiently digest that richness. Meanwhile, sour citrus and refreshing herbs offset the heating quality of the spices. Adding noodles, vegetables and mushrooms to the stock means that this dish is very satisfying – it's a classic one-pot meal.

Variations

The variations to this dish are legion. For a start, it can be cooked with all manner of seasonal vegetables, whether they are root vegetables or leafy greens.

Similarly, the fresh herbs that are used can be your favourites or those that are looking particularly perky in the garden at the time. Lemon or lime can provide citrus flavours.

Try experimenting with spices and other ingredients. Coriander, cumin, allspice and paprika all go well with chicken, while adding a bit of coconut cream gives it a bit of a South-East Asian feel.

Otherwise, your broth can follow classical lines as with the two examples given below.

Aromatic chicken broth with noodles

In essence, this describes a typical European soup. It is a light dish, deriving its richness from highly digestible chicken meat and stock, and it is therefore well suited to hot and dry summer days. Its flavours are moderate with no intense spicy ingredients. Aromatic flavours come from onion and fresh herbs such as basil, marjoram, chives, chervil and parsley. Bitterness is also important in this sort of dish to counter the effect of hot weather, so select from watercress, chicory, celery, dandelion, rocket and chard to enhance the broth.

Spicy chicken broth with noodles

Spicy chicken broth is a typical dish of the humid areas of South-East Asia. There are great regional variations on this theme but two key principles remain the same: lightness for the heat of the climate, and spice to cut through the obstructiveness of the humidity. A typical example of this is a Sichuanese chicken broth which is founded on the zingy Sichuanese pepper and lots of fiery chilli. Such is the spicy strength of this dish that it brings on copious sweating, another mechanism that is thought to help with overcoming intense heat and humidity.

When I was studying in the traditional hospital in Chengdu, the capital of Sichuan, many of the doctors said that things had gone to far. The strength of spice in the local cuisine was damaging people's health, and it is certainly true that these spices can have an inflammatory effect on the gut.

So, when we get hot and humid weather here in Britain, it is a good idea to add some chilli and Sichuan pepper to your chicken noodle broth... but not too much!

Mushroom risotto

Serves 4

Ingredients

1 tbsp dried porcini mushrooms
olive oil
1 onion, chopped
2 garlic cloves, finely chopped
225 g chestnut mushrooms, sliced
350 g arborio rice or pearled spelt
150 ml dry white wine
1.2 litres hot best vegetable stock
handful chopped fresh parsley
25 g butter
salt and freshly ground black pepper
freshly grated parmesan, to serve

Method

Soak the mushrooms in a little hot water for 10 minutes. In a heavy-based pan fry the onion and garlic in a little olive oil for around 2 minutes. Add the chestnut mushrooms and cook for a further 2 minutes. Stir in the rice and make sure it is well coated with the cooking oil. Pour in the wine, simmer and stir until it has all been absorbed. Begin to add the stock, a ladleful at a time, maintaining a simmer and adding a fresh ladle of stock as the last one is absorbed. Continue adding the stock in this way until it has all been absorbed and the rice is tender or to your liking. Roughly chop the soaked mushrooms, add those, the soaking water, parsley and butter to the risotto and stir through. Put a lid on the dish and allow it to sit for just a few minutes before serving with the grated parmesan.

Any dish that uses mushrooms as this one does is medicinal, such is their nutritional value. In this case the mushrooms form the basis for a light dish suited to cold, dry winter weather, suffused as it is with the aromatics of the onion, garlic, parsley and pepper that warm and stimulate circulation in the gut. Balancing this expansiveness is the astringency of the wine, while the bitterness of the parsley adds depth of flavour and stimulates secretion.

Variations

Arborio rice is not grown in Britain but pearled spelt is and makes a nice local alternative for risottos. You should be able to get it in a good health-food store. Spelt is richer than rice and will require more spice for balance. This can be provided with some extra black pepper or paprika. Spice can be used to compensate for extra dampness in the climate too.

If you are eating this dish in summer, add some bitter greens such as dandelion, chicory, rocket or nasturtium. The bitterness helps to cool the warmth of the aromatics.

Nasturtium, chicken and pesto salad

Ingredients

leftover chicken or sautéed chicken breast
pesto
nasturtium flowers
lemon juice
black pepper
watercress

Method

Cover the chicken with generous amounts of pesto, then squeeze on a little lemon juice and black pepper. Top with a few nasturtium flowers and sprigs of watercress. Serve with macaroni or gnocchi while it is still hot.

This is light summer food at its simplest. Like all of this diet's salads, its major components, chicken and macaroni or gnocchi, are cooked, so that even in the hottest and driest weather much of the work is done for our digestive systems by the cooking process. Accompanying these ingredients is a little extra sweetness from the olive oil of the pesto. Basil (in the pesto), black pepper and the watercress provide spicy aromatics, lemon juice, a refreshing sourness to counter the heat of the weather, and nasturtium flowers, a zingy bitterness, again ideally suited to compensating for hot weather.

Variations

The best way to add variety to this dish is by making your

own pesto. Olive oil can be substituted with rapeseed or hemp oil and basil replaced with parsley or coriander.

Nasturtium leaves can be used as well as the flowers and other bitter salad greens used instead of, or alongside, the watercress.

Digestion-friendly pancakes

One egg's worth of mixture produces roughly two pancakes.

Ingredients

1 egg
2 heaped tbsp barley/buckwheat flour (wholegrain preferred)
^{1}/2 mug oat/almond/rice milk

Method

Put the ingredients in a bowl and use a hand blender until they are thoroughly mixed and there are no lumps.

Cook the pancakes with a knob of butter.

Pancakes are delicious and particularly popular with kids. And I can reassure you that, after years of testing on my children and other people's, this recipe is also up to the mark when it comes to taste and satisfaction.

As traditional mixes combine wheat flour with cow's milk, they are particularly heavy and inhibit motility. With this recipe I substitute these bogey ingredients with other flours, which nourish symbionts and are much lighter than wheat, and milk alternatives that are lighter than cow's milk. Bingo – the richness of the egg is offset by the lightness of the other two ingredients. This makes a much more digestible pancake with no compromise in flavour. Using a wholemeal flour adds the benefit of extra fibre and nutrients and creates a deeper, nuttier taste.

Note that in this case I do not recommend soy milk.

Currently, there are valid doubts over the health properties of unfermented soy products which need further clarification; until I receive it I cannot confidently suggest soy milk as a substitute for cow's milk.

Variations

The French use buckwheat flour in their *galette*, a traditional type of pancake. This grain nourishes digestion, as do others such as millet, rye and maize. All of these flours can be used instead of wheat in a pancake recipe – it is just a question of what sort of taste you enjoy.

When it comes to the alternative "milks" – like rice, oat and almond – watch out for added sugar.

Spices can also be added to pancake mix. A favourite at home is lightly toasted fennel seeds, a wonderful stimulant for motility when combined with this relatively rich food.

Spicy scrambled eggs

Serves 2

Ingredients

4 organic eggs, beaten
4 spring onions or 1 red onion, finely chopped
2 cloves garlic, finely chopped or minced
1 green chilli, finely chopped – optional
½ tsp garam masala
½ tsp mustard seeds
¼ tsp turmeric
4 medium tomatoes, chopped
small handful coriander

Method

Fry the onions, garlic and chilli (if using) for about 5 minutes until the onions are soft and translucent. Add the spices and cook for a further 3 minutes. Add the chopped tomatoes and continue to cook until they start to break up. Pour in the eggs and continue to stir until they are cooked to your liking, adding the coriander about a minute before serving.

Scrambled eggs are convenient and nutritious. But they are particularly rich, which is why they've had a bad press over the years, blamed for cholesterol trouble and high levels of allergy and intolerance.

The picture would be different if we combined them intelligently with a good mix of aromatic vegetables, herbs and spices to stimulate digestion. Which is precisely what this recipe does, with garam masala, mustard seeds, turmeric and chilli to cut through the richness and stimulate secretion. Garlic and onion boost motility to get the gut moving. Because of the intensity of the spices, we use the sourness of the tomato and the freshness of the coriander to cool and mellow the dish.

Variations

In this recipe, the scrambled eggs have been taken down the spicy route to compensate for their richness. But not everyone gets on with strong spices, in which case you might prefer herby eggs. If you have them in your garden, pick a handful of fresh aromatic herbs, chop them up and combine them with some black pepper. Particularly good herbs to combine with eggs are sweet cicely, tarragon and thyme.

Tuna, fennel and bean salad

Serves 4

Ingredients

1 small head fennel, fronds removed
1 medium red onion, quartered
2 cloves garlic
2 x 400 g cans cannellini beans, drained and rinsed
extra-virgin olive oil
juice of half a lemon
handful fresh flatleaf parsley leaves, chopped
2 x 200 g cans tuna steak in spring water or olive oil, drained
60 g black olives (pitted, if preferred)

Method

Trim and quarter the fennel and reserve the fronds. Put in a roasting dish with the quartered onion and a couple of garlic cloves. I usually do several of each at one time to save time and energy. Give them a generous drizzle of olive oil and bake in the oven at around 180°C for 20 minutes.

Slice the baked onion and fennel finely and place in a bowl with the beans and parsley. Whisk two tablespoons of olive oil with the lemon juice; stir it in the salad. Leave to stand for a few minutes. Meanwhile, drain the tins of tuna and gently stir the fish and the olives into the salad. Serve with the reserved fennel fronds to garnish.

This is the ideal working lunch for cold, dry winter's days. Digestion is assisted by the fact that the salad is largely cooked. In addition, mild aromatics from the fennel, onion, garlic and parsley, stimulate gut motility and secretion; and olive oil and tuna add richness, balanced by a little lemon juice, to make the dish sustaining through the cold winter afternoon.

Variations

If you're at home or can get to a frying pan, it is just as good, and perhaps more convenient, to fry off the garlic, fennel and onion with olive oil for 10 minutes, rather than baking it.

You can also add whatever fresh herbs you might have to hand, such as rosemary, marjoram, basil, coriander or tarragon. These add wonderful aromatic depth to the dish. You can, of course, also add a little extra spice such as some deseeded chilli or cumin seeds.

Warm potato salad

Ingredients

potatoes – new, salad or boiling
a small handful fresh mint
a small handful chives/spring onion
a few capers
mayonnaise

Method

Add the mayonnaise to the potatoes when they are still warm with the mint, chives and capers. Gently mix it all together.

Potato salad is one of the perpetual disappointments of the British summer. Bland, claggy and cold, it's just not appetising. But this *warm* potato salad is. Because it is warm, the mayonnaise melts a bit and the raw flavours of the herbs soften and blend.

Meanwhile, because of the mint, capers, chives and pepper, there are plenty of aromatic flavours to stimulate the appetite, assist motility and relieve the richness of the mayonnaise. The sour lemon juice enhances this effect to make a classic mix of sour and aromatic flavours.

Variations

Because the basic ingredients of this recipe – potatoes and mayonnaise –are bland, a wide range of flavours, particularly fresh aromatic herbs can be added. Try marjoram, tarragon or basil. Or a teaspoon of mustard.

As a tasty alternative, what about adding some finely chopped red onion, caramelised in a little olive oil?

Aromatic mussels with cider and bacon

Serves 2

Ingredients

1 kg mussels, scrubbed and debearded
1 tbsp olive oil
knob of unsalted butter
100 g streaky bacon, roughly chopped
1 bunch spring onions sliced
2 sprigs thyme, leaves removed
1 bay leaf
250 ml medium-sweet cider
1 tsp wholegrain mustard
2-3 tbsp crème fraîche
seasoning
2 handfuls chopped flat-leaf parsley
a pinch of chilli flakes

Method

Discard any mussels that don't close when tapped on a hard surface. In a large heavy bottomed saucepan, heat the olive oil and butter until the butter begins to foam. Add the bacon and cook for 4 minutes, then stir in the spring onions. Add the thyme and the bay leaf and continue to cook for 2 minutes. Turn the heat right up and add the mussels, giving the pan a good shake and turning the mussels over in the cooking juices. Pour in the cider and stir in the mustard. Put a lid on the pan and allow it to steam for 3 minutes giving the pan a good shake every minute. Remove the lid and discard any mussels that haven't opened. Stir in the crème fraîche and warm through for a further 30 seconds. Stir in the parsley and chilli flakes, season and serve.

Mussels are a constitutional tonic food, full of minerals and nutrients, and therefore great to eat, but they are very rich. Similarly, the other rich ingredients – butter, bacon, crème fraîche –are variously fatty and sweet and therefore delicious, but they all tend to cause sluggish motility in the gut, just like the mussels.

It is therefore very important to combine these rich ingredients with aromatic, moving and dispersing herbs and spices to stimulate secretion and get the gut moving. Spring onion, parsley, thyme, bay, mustard and a little bit of chilli do just such a job, warming and stimulating the intestines. As a counterbalance to this strong stimulus, cider is sour and astringent, calming the excesses of the spice and creating balance in the dish.

Variations

The mussel season starts in September and continues through the winter, so this is a cold-weather dish. If you find that the weather is particularly bracing, you may prefer to use white wine instead of cider as it is not quite as astringent. Even less astringent are rice wine and sherry which also go well with mussels.

Using coconut cream instead of crème fraîche and coriander leaf instead of parsley takes the dish in a South-East Asian direction.

Basic stir-fry

Serves 4

Ingredients

300 g fresh beef, filleted chicken or tofu
2 cm fresh ginger root
1 clovegarlic
1 chilli, deseeded
6 spring onions
soy sauce
5 tbsp sunflower oil
2 handfuls mushrooms
2 handfuls seasonal veg
2 handfuls seasonal greens
2 tsp toasted sesame oil
a handful chopped fresh basil

Method

Heat half the sunflower oil in a wok. Add the meat or tofu and sear it. If using chicken make sure it is clearly cooked through but still tender. Remove the meat or tofu from the wok and add the rest of the sunflower oil. Add the veg, mushroom and spices to the wok. Heat and stir for 3 minutes. Add the meat and cook for a further 30 seconds. Remove from the heat and stir in the basil and the toasted sesame oil. Add soy sauce at the end to taste.

There was a time in Britain when just about everything, including lettuce, was cooked. Though things have changed and we now eat lots of raw and unseasonal fruit and veg, this iconic Chinese dish illustrates that elsewhere in the world raw food is still considered crude and hard to digest.

The stir-fry works on the basis that even a little bit of cooking "opens up" our food, breaking it down enough to give our digestive systems a helping hand. It also allows flavours to mellow, mingle and mature.

In this recipe there are some of the stalwarts of the Chinese kitchen cupboard: chilli, garlic, ginger, spring onion and soy sauce. And all of these help digestion in their way. Garlic, chilli and ginger help it through strongly stimulating gut circulation, motility and secretion so that the lightly cooked vegetables can be easily broken down and absorbed. The spring onion adds strong aromatic to the same effect while the soy sauce adds savoury depth to stimulate appetite.

Adding a little bit of toasted sesame oil at the end of cooking is a good trick with stir fries, especially when cooking with tofu. It adds richness, especially in the cold months.

Variations

Stir-fry has exceptional variety as a dish, just about any vegetable, mushroom and meat can be used. The key thing is the principles that underlie the dish: light cooking to enhance digestion and develop flavours, and the right herbs and spices to assist digestion. Try adding Chinese five-spice and experiment with seasonal leafy herbs as we have with basil in this recipe.

Ceviche

Serves about 3

Ingredients

500 g fresh sea bass fillet, cut into 1 cm pieces
60 ml freshly squeezed lemon juice
60 ml freshly squeezed lime juice
½ a small red onion, finely diced
1 fresh tomato chopped and seeded
1 mild chilli, seeded and finely chopped
1 tsp salt
¼ tsp freshly ground black pepper
1 small pinch cayenne pepper
¼ handful chopped dill

Method

Place the fish, onion, tomato, chilli, black pepper, cayenne pepper and dill in a ceramic, glass or porcelain dish. Pour the lemon and lime juice over them and mix it all up well. Leave in the fridge for about 3 hours, gently mixing every hour. Do not leave for more than two hours or the fish will lose too much of its firmness.

Ceviche is made with immense variety of fish throughout much of Latin America. It is a dish designed to match their hot, dry climate, composed as it is of raw ingredients with a predominant sour, refreshing taste. The sourness comes from the acidity of the lemon and lime juice which does the "cooking", as the acid reacts with the proteins of the fish to break them down. Nonetheless, a dish with so many raw ingredients takes some digesting, especially since the citrus acid makes it so astringent. Therefore the recipe contains significant expansive spice in the chilli, cayenne pepper and black pepper, all of which strongly stimulate motility and secretion. Sweet is also an expansive flavour, provided in this case by the tomato and onion, although some ceviche recipes incorporate a little sugar too.

Dill is included, as a mild aromatic component redolent of the British summer and a marvellous companion to fish.

Variations

This dish, despite its multitude of regional and cultural variations, first and foremost is only suitable for the hottest and driest British summers. When they come along, it's perfect food!

Some people struggle with really acidic food, and one way to compensate for this is to add a little sugar as I have already mentioned. Some diced mango, whose sweetness and flavour profile perfectly matches the other ingredients, is also a great addition.

Kedgeree

Serves 2-4

Ingredients

2 eggs
6 spring onions, finely chopped
2 bay leaves
115 g butter
1 clove garlic finely chopped
680 g un-dyed smoked haddock (it's worth a couple
of minutes to pin bone it)
170 g basmati rice
2 heaped tsp curry powder (or 1 tsp each of
ground coriander, cumin and turmeric)
juice of 1 lemon
2 handfuls chopped coriander
a small finger of grated ginger

Method

Hard-boil the eggs for 8 to 10 minutes, remove and plunge in cold water to stop the cooking process.

Put the haddock in a frying pan with the 2 bay leaves, cover with water and simmer for around 5 minutes.

Cook the basmati rice in water for 10 minutes and drain.

Now melt the butter in a pan on a low heat. Slowly cook the spring onions and garlic until translucent. Add the curry powder or spices and cook for a further 3 minutes. Add the rice to the pan and stir through with the lemon juice, gently warming it through. Fold the fish and coriander in until it is all nicely warm and ready to serve.

This is a seriously tasty dish! But eggs, butter and smoked haddock take some digesting.

Smoking any type of food is a way of preserving it. It partially cooks it and changes its chemical structure to make it harder to digest, not only for bacteria and moulds, but for us too. This means that although the smoky flavour is delightful, we need lots of sour and aromatic ingredients to help the fish to break down once we've eaten it. The same principle applies to the butter and the eggs.

Sourness is provided by the lemon, while aromatic flavours come from ginger, garlic, spring onion, coriander, cumin and turmeric. Turmeric also provides bitterness to strongly stimulate motility, and coriander leaf plays an increasingly familiar role here as it balances out the heating action of the spices.

Variations

The sour and bitter flavours of this dish can be enhanced by adding lemon zest. Parsley will add bitterness and boost the refreshing action of the coriander leaf. More bitterness is great if you are prone to a sluggish bowel.

If you like a bit more spice, paprika and mustard seeds are mild and combine well with the other spices. And you could try cooking the rice with saffron.

Finely diced carrot and peas can be added to bring sweetness the dish, a particularly child-friendly ruse!

Lemon chicken

Serves 4-6

Ingredients

1 large chicken, jointed into 8–10 pieces
olive oil
1 head garlic, halved horizontally
thyme sprigs
splash of sherry vinegar
2 tbsp dark soy sauce
3 tbsp honey
1 lemon, finely sliced (ideally with a mandolin)
a handful flat-leaf parsley, finely chopped
seasoning

Method

Season the chicken with salt and pepper and heat the olive oil in a large frying pan. Brown the chicken pieces in batches with the garlic and thyme for 2 or 3 minutes on each side.

Return all the chicken to the pan, add the sherry vinegar and bubble until reduced by half. Drizzle over the soy sauce and honey and shake the pan to mix.

Pour in a good splash of hot water and add the lemon slices. Let the liquid reduce down until syrupy, around 10 minutes. Check to make sure the chicken is cooked through. Sprinkle with the parsley.

Another chicken dish! But I wanted to include this one because it's nutritious and so easy to cook. The ingredients provide a classic balanced combination of all of the flavours – sweet (chicken and honey), sour (lemon and vinegar), salty/savoury (soy sauce), bitter (lemon zest and pith and parsley) and aromatic/pungent (garlic, thyme, parsley and seasoning). Served with rice and some steamed greens, lemon chicken is incredible easy to digest.

Variations

This simple recipe can be whipped up in no time, but if you're really pressed, don't bother jointing the chicken. Just brown the chicken skin all over in a wok, bung in the other ingredients, pop on the lid and leave it to cook.

If you have more time, get a chicken with giblets and boil up a small stock on the side with a couple of bay leaves. This stock, added to the sauce and reduced, adds lots of nutrition and depth of flavour.

Indeed, with a litre of stock, the recipe can be converted into a one-pot meal, with root vegetables and fresh herbs placed around the chicken in a big pan or wok. You could also add a bit more spice. Smoked paprika is particularly good, creating a lovely mellow depth of flavour.

Salmon and caper fishcakes

Serves 1

Ingredients

tin of wild salmon or grilled salmon steak
1 tsp capers, rinsed and drained
120 g mashed potato
bag of watercress
3 big pinches cayenne pepper
3 tbsp olive oil
semolina
mayonnaise

Method

If using tinned salmon drain it well in a sieve, pressing it down with the back of a spoon. Then place it in a bowl with the capers and potato.

Chop three quarters of the watercress and add a large tablespoon to the bowl. Add some salt and the cayenne pepper and mix everything well together.

Sprinkle some semolina onto a plate, then divide the salmon mix into six. Shape them into rounds using your hands, coating each one fully with semolina.

Heat the oil in a wok or large frying pan and when it is very hot, add the fishcakes and cook them briefly – about 2 minutes on each side.

Serve with remaining watercress and mayonnaise.

The lightness of this dish makes it ideal for hot and humid weather, as it is not particularly rich and fatty while the spice of the pepper, combined with the pungent bitterness of watercress strongly stimulates appetite and motility. Little wonder that it is such an iconic dish in the humid tropics. It is also cheap; an ideal way to use up leftover fish and mashed potato.

Variations

In drier hot weather, refreshing aromatic herbs such as mint, coriander and marjoram can be added to the mix. If it is more humid and damp, try using a little sweet chilli sauce as a condiment.

In colder weather, more richness is required which can be provided by adding extra mayonnaise.

Sausage casserole

Serves 4

Ingredients

8 medium-sized good-quality sausages (two per person), pork, beef and lamb sausages are all suitable.
1 medium-sized onion chopped
4 shallots, roughly chopped
2 crushed garlic cloves
2 medium-sized potatoes peeled and diced into cubes
2 red peppers, sliced
400 g tin chopped tomatoes
$1/2$ pint chicken stock
400 g tin lentils
1 tbsp of cider vinegar
1 sprig chopped rosemary
knob of butter

Method

Melt the butter in a large heavy bottomed casserole dish on a medium heat on top of the stove. Pierce the sausages then brown all over. Remove from the dish, then put the onions, shallots and garlic in. Cook slowly for about 5 minutes or until they start to become tender.

Add the cubed potatoes and fry for a further 5 minutes, taking care not to burn the onions and garlic. Add the chicken stock gradually, stir well and add the sausages. Add half the rosemary and all of the other ingredients.

The liquid should cover the sausages, and reduce down during cooking by as much as half.

Continue to cook on the stove for a few minutes, gradually increasing the heat until the pot is simmering. Taste the sauce: if it's too acidic, add a pinch or two of brown sugar. Cook uncovered for about an hour in the oven at 180°C.

Remove from the oven, garnish with the remaining rosemary and serve with fresh broad beans and rice or polenta.

This is the ideal winter dish. It is not only thrifty, combining cheap meat and pulses, it is also nourishing and filling. This sort of rich aromatic food is perfectly suited to cold and damp weather, underpinned as it is by pungent, expansive onions, garlic and rosemary, with the sourness of vinegar to cut through the fat and richness.

Variations

You could add more spice or more aromatic herbs, particularly if you're not cooking for children!

This would be particularly beneficial if using pork sausages, as they are so obstructive to motility. Good herbs to add are a classic bouquet garni of bay, thyme and sage. Good spices are paprika, star anise and mustard seeds.

More complex recipes

Grilled or barbecued sardines with salsa

Serves 4

Ingredients

8 sardines, cleaned and gutted
3 tbsp olive oil
2 sprigs thyme leaves picked
2 cloves of garlic, finely chopped
sea salt and ground pepper

Method

Combine the olive oil, garlic, thyme and seasoning. Rub the mixture all over the sardines, inside and out. If barbecuing, then place them in a fish basket and grill them over hot coals for a couple of minutes on each side until they are crisp and bubbling. Or place them under a hot grill for 3 to 4 minutes each side until the skin begins to darken.

Serve with the tomato salsa.

The salsa

Ingredients

250 g fresh tomatoes, finely chopped
1 small onion, finely chopped

3 mild chillies, finely chopped
small handful of coriander, finely chopped
salt to taste
lime juice to taste
1 tbsp water

Method

Mix all the ingredients together in a bowl. Best left for at least a couple of hours to infuse.

Sardines are in season in the UK during the summer months, and they are cheap and delicious barbecued. Consequently, this an ideal summer dish. In terms of our diet, the main principle that this recipe demonstrates is the use of an aromatic rub and a spicy sour salsa to help digest the rich oily meat of the fish. These stimulate gut motility and bile secretion, helping to avoid tiring sluggishness. The added benefit of this approach is that is offers a broad and deliciously appetising flavour profile.

Variations

The same method can be applied to other fatty fish such as mackerel, herring (both of which are in season during the summer) and sprats. These fish are lovely when grilled or barbecued. Indeed, it makes sense to be prepared and have a nice salsa on standby in the fridge throughout the summer months.

Boiled ham hocks with pease pudding

Serves 4-6

Ingredients for the ham hocks

4 fresh ham hocks
2 onions, roughly chopped
2 carrots, roughly chopped
2 sticks celery, roughly chopped
4 or 5 black peppercorns, whole
3 cloves
2 bay leaves

For the peas pudding

350g yellow slit peas, soaked overnight
1 onion, fined diced
1 garlic clove, finely chopped
a small tied bunch of thyme, rosemary, bay and sage.
butter and seasoning

Method

Line a bowl with a square of muslin cloth. Rinse the soaked peas and mix them with the garlic, onion and herbs. Place them in the lined bowl and tightly twist and tie the cloth to make a parcel. Reserve the butter and seasoning.

Put the muslin parcel, ham hocks and all the other ingredients in a deep saucepan. Cover with cold water, bring to the boil and simmer for around 2 to 3 hours until the meat is wonderfully tender and falling off the bone. Scrape the pease pudding from the cloth, remove the herbs and mash with the reserved butter and seasoning.

Additions

Add whole baby carrots, small leeks and a fennel bulb half an hour before the end of cooking. Serve these as an accompaniment. Use the strained stock as gravy. Serve the dish with English mustard.

The combination of rich, salty or preserved meat with pulses is popular throughout the world. Think mutton and lentils, cassoulet, or bacon and peas. This is the original poor man's hearty meal and uses the principle of combining rich, flavoursome meat with pulses to marry flavour, fat and richness with the bulk and protein of the beans.

And it's cheap.

True to this diet's principles, a superb organic ham hock can be bought for a few pounds. Once it has been boiled up, the goodness has passed from the bones and the marrow to the broth, resulting in a wonderful tasty, nutritious dish.

Boiling also enhances the digestibility of the hock as it disperses its richness into the broth, in contrast to baking or roasting which concentrates the fats in the meat, exaggerating the work that the bile salts, digestive enzymes and symbionts have to do to break it down.

It thus employs precisely the same elegant nutritional principles as any bone stock; the balanced combination of celery, carrot and onion together with other aromatic spices (cloves and peppercorns) and herbs (garlic, thyme, rosemary, bay and sage).

Using a range of herbs broadens the health-enhancing effect of the dish; bay, sage and thyme are all bitter so stimulate bowel movement in response to preserved meat, while rosemary specifically counters the symptom of trapped wind – a particular problem when consuming large amounts of beans!

Variations

Suffice it to say that there are plenty of recipes along these lines out there in traditional cuisines around the world. They might be with mutton, pork, duck or beef and a range of pulses from lentils to haricot beans. All of them provide nutritious, delicious and cheap food.

From this diet's perspective, there are a few issues that are important. The first is to take time to cook the dish in the first place, as the preparation of the beans and the bone stock is time-intensive. The second is to use plenty of really fresh herbs to refresh and balance out the effects of the spices, broaden the flavour profile and raise the aromatic oil content of the dish. And finally, the spices are important to cut through the fatty intensity of the meat.

Cassoulet

Serves 8+ and keeps well in the fridge

Ingredients

5 tbsp olive oil
5 belly pork ribs
100 g bacon pieces
3 cloves, crushed
2 onions, finely chopped
3 garlic cloves, finely chopped
1 carrot, diced
2 celery sticks, finely chopped
1 leek, finely sliced
1 litre chicken stock
1 tin plum tomatoes, finely chopped
1 tbsp of lemon juice
3 tins white haricot beans, drained
(or 600 g beans, cooked from dry)
4 confit duck legs
4 bay leaves and a handful each of chopped thyme and sage
salt and black pepper
a handful of chopped flat-leaf parsley

Method

Heat the olive oil in a pan and add the belly pork ribs. Fry the pork until it is browned all over, then remove it from the pan. Now add the bacon, cloves, onions, garlic, carrot, celery and leek to the pan and fry until the onion is translucent. Return the pork to the pan with these ingredients and add the lemon juice, stock, tomatoes, bay, thyme, sage and duck, bring to the boil and simmer for 1 ½ hours with the lid off so that the sauce thickens over time. Add the beans and simmer for a further 30 minutes. Add salt, pepper and flat-leaf parsley to taste. It can then be served hot, although due to its high fat content the cassoulet is often allowed to cool and, once a layer of fat has risen to the top and solidified, it is skimmed off to reduce the fatty, cloying nature of the dish. It is then reheated to serve.

Cassoulet derives its name from the French word "cassole" which is the name of the earthenware ovenproof dish in which this type of food is normally cooked. It is a classic and appears in many guises, featuring other rich meats such a pork, mutton, goose, sausages and pancetta. But they all exist within a framework that combines fatty meat with beans, creating a nutritious, sustaining but not over-rich concoction. "Peasant food", if you like, although such is the cultural depth of cassoulet that it can be found on all menus regardless of class.

This recipe is typical, with a good chicken bone stock and pork ribs thrown in to add extra nutrition. Traditionally, it's a winter food, but a *French* winter, which is typically drier than ours, especially in the mountains where it gets very cold. That is why its flavour profile is predominantly aromatic rather than spicy; the onion, garlic, bay, thyme and sage are just about enough to stimulate gut motility in the face of this hearty fare. The aromatics are helped in this task by sourness (lemon, tomato) and bitterness (celery, sage).

Otherwise this is first and foremost a naturally sweet dish with beans, onions, carrot, leek and meat cooking down over time to produce a deep enriching flavour that suits our energy-hungry winter metabolisms.

Variations

The internet, long-standing chefs and classic French cookbooks all have multiple versions of cassoulet. For our purposes, the key is to embrace its fundamentals: sweet aromatic veg, lovely rich meat and bones, a good stock, fresh aromatic herbs and lots of beans. For damper winter days it is worth experimenting with more intense flavours, especially spice. Particularly good are allspice, aniseed, caraway, clove, fennel, juniper, mustard seed, paprika and star anise, although these need to be matched with the choice of meat. The same effect can be achieved by adding a spicy sausage such as chorizo or merguez.

Of course it is also great to use different types of bean, particularly other pale, soft and sweet varieties such as butter beans.

Chicken chasseur

Serves 4

Ingredients

1 tsp olive oil
25 g butter
4 chicken legs
1 onion, chopped
2 garlic cloves , finely chopped
200 g chestnut mushrooms
2 thyme sprigs
225 ml red wine
2 tbsp tomato purée
500 ml best chicken stock

Method

In a large heavy-bottomed casserole pan, heat the olive oil and half the butter. When the butter is bubbling, fry the chicken on both sides until browned. Remove the chicken, add the rest of the butter to the pan and begin to soften the onion. When the onion is translucent and soft, add the garlic and then the mushrooms and the thyme. Continue to cook for a further 3 or 4 minutes before adding the wine and the tomato purée. Once this has begun to reduce after around 5 minutes then add the chicken back to the pan before adding the stock. Put a lid on the pan and cook gently over a low heat for around an hour. Remove the chicken legs and keep warm. Reduce the sauce over a high heat for a few minutes before serving.

Based on a 400-year-old recipe, "hunter's chicken" is

wonderfully sustaining and therefore suited to the relatively cold British climate. We should feel free to eat it through the autumn, winter and spring.

It is rich (chicken, chicken stock, butter, olive oil and wine), and nourishing (chestnut mushrooms), but not strongly spiced, relying instead on aromatic flavours from onion, garlic and thyme to stimulate motility and secretion.

Variations

The dish has only small amounts of bitterness (thyme) and sour (tomato), which firmly establishes it as a cold-weather dish. It's lack of spice also makes it as a predominantly dry-weather dish. With damper weather, we should ideally give it some more oomph, perhaps through adding mustard seeds or extra black pepper.

Chicken curry

Serves 4

Ingredients

4 chicken thighs, preferably free-range or organic
3 tbsp coconut oil or ghee
1 tsp yellow or brown mustard seeds
1 large onion, sliced
3 garlic cloves, finely sliced
1 x 400 ml canned coconut milk

For the marinade:
1 tsp paprika
½ tsp ground turmeric or 2 cm piece of turmeric root
1½ tbsp ground coriander
1 tsp ground cumin
1 tsp cayenne pepper
1 tbsp lemon juice
½ tsp raw sea salt
75 ml water

Method

Mix all the marinade ingredients together and add the chicken pieces. They are best left to marinate for at least an hour but preferably overnight.

Heat the oil or ghee in a deep frying pan and add the mustard seeds. When they start to pop and jump about in the pan, add the onion and garlic. Cook until they're soft and translucent, then add the chicken and any extra paste from the marinade. Fry over a gentle heat for about

8 minutes, turning the chicken occasionally. Then add the coconut milk. Increase the heat slightly and bring to a simmer. Cook for a further 10-12 minutes until the sauce has thickened slightly and serve with rice or flat bread.

There are many chicken curries around, but compared with typical restaurant or takeaway offerings which either blow your head off or sit like a lead weight in your stomach, this recipe shapes up very nicely indeed. It is light, with a balanced mix of spices. Not too hot, with some lovely bitterness from the turmeric.

In terms of the British climate, this dish can be eaten all year round, with the main ingredients chicken and coconut milk providing just the right level of richness and digestibility.

Variations

Earlier in the book we refer to this as a summer dish; light but with spices to cut through the dampness of the climate. It can easily be made more summery with the addition of more refreshing flavours, in particular bitter, sour and cooling aromatics. For bitter, use steamed greens; for sour, add extra lemon juice or lemon zest; and for cooling aromatics, choose fresh coriander leaf. Lovely.

Dal

Serves 3

Ingredients

cooking fat – coconut oil (if vegan)
ghee/clarified butter (if vegetarian)
1 medium yellow onion, quartered
25 g grated coconut/coconut cream
3 cloves garlic, sliced
2 chillies, deseeded and finely diced
1 tbsp fresh ginger root, minced
2 tsp garam masala
1 tsp ground cumin
1/2 tsp cinnamon
1/4 tsp turmeric
1/4 tsp ground coriander
240 ml light chicken or vegetable stock or water
400 g tomatoes, diced
230 g pumpkin, peeled and diced
360 g cooked black-eyed peas
70 g spinach, chopped
some finely shredded mint

Method

Combine onion, coconut, garlic, chillies, ginger, garam masala, cumin, cinnamon, salt, turmeric, coriander and 3 tbsp (45ml) stock in a blender. Purée mixture to a paste, scraping down the sides of the blender as necessary.

Heat the cooking fat in a large saucepan, and then add the spice paste and cook, stirring often, for 10 minutes.

Add remaining stock, tomatoes and pumpkin. Cook over medium heat, stirring often, until pumpkin is just tender: about 20 minutes.

Mix in black-eyed peas and spinach. Continue to cook, stirring often, for 5 more minutes. Remove from heat. Taste and adjust seasonings; stir in the mint just before serving.

This is a spice-heavy dish that often forms part of a vegetarian menu. Interestingly, since it is a vegetarian stalwart, from this diet's perspective its value lies not so much in its spices as in its cooking fat and protein content. This is because vegetarian diets often lack necessary richness, the sort of richness supplied by coconut oil or ghee and beans.

Ghee and coconut oil are both high in short-chain saturated fats, the sort that are easy to digest and strongly nourish blood, membranes and the nervous system. Because they are saturated, they are perfect for frying spices, maintaining their chemical structure even at high temperature. Meanwhile, beans are a great source of vegetarian protein.

On their own, the combination of the saturated fat and the beans would present something of a digestive challenge. But not with the plethora of herbs and spices that accompany them in this dish. Tthe standard Asian pungent and spicy ingredients onion, garlic, ginger and chilli cut through the fat and stimulate secretion and motility.

Garam masala, also used in this recipe, literally translates as "hot mixture" but is better translated as "mixture of spices" since most of the spices involved tend to be mellow in flavour: cloves, cinnamon, nutmeg, cardamom, cumin and coriander seeds. The ingredients of garam masala vary according to the region of origin and the taste of the chef. So have a look at the packet when you buy the pre-prepared stuff in case you have a flavour preference or don't like very spicy food as some brands will include chilli.

Of course, true to the principles of this diet, we should be making our own garam masala by grinding up our own personal combination of whole spices, releasing the full potential of the aromatic oils and fresh flavours.

Variations

The recipe, as we have it here, is a complex one, with lots of spicy and aromatic ingredients. But it doesn't have to be. If you don't like very spicy food, leave out the chilli and cut down on garlic. Or you can make your own garam masala with just a few mild spices like cumin, coriander, cardamom and star anise.

Similarly, you may enjoy adding different refreshing and cooling ingredients beyond the sour tomatoes and aromatic mint that we have here. How about fresh coriander leaf (aromatic), lemon or sorrel (sour), or spinach (sweet and bitter)?

Other dal recipes include different pulses such as green, black or yellow lentils and split peas. All of these mush down nicely and are delicious.

Falafel

Serves 1–2

Ingredients

1 400 g tin chickpeas, drained and rinsed, or 200 g dried
chick peas, soaked overnight
1 small onion, finely chopped
2 cloves garlic, finely chopped
1 small bunch parsley, stalks removed, leaves finely
chopped
1 small bunch coriander, stalks removed, leaves finely
chopped
1 tsp ground cumin
¼ tsp chilli flakes (optional)
2-3 tbsp plain flour
lemon juice

Method

Combine the chickpeas, onion and garlic in a food proc-
essor. Add the herbs, cumin, chilli and a small pinch of sea
salt, and pulse to a coarse paste. Add the flour a little at a
time until the mixture comes together roughly in a ball. Put
it into a bowl, cover and refrigerate for a couple of hours.

Pre-heat the oven to 200°C. Roll the falafel mix into
golf-ball-sized rounds. Line a baking tray with lightly oiled
baking parchment, line up the balls so they don't touch and
bake for around 20 minutes.

Squeeze on fresh lemon juice before eating. Serve with a
cooked grain and lightly cooked vegetables or some bitter
leaves and a spicy pickle. Tahini (sesame paste) thinned with

water and lemon juice is also a delicious accompaniment.

Falafel is an ancient dish illustrating a key principle of traditional cuisine. A bland, fibrous stable (chickpeas) is overlaid by intense and balanced flavours to make it appetising and easy to digest. In this case, sweet (chickpeas, onion), aromatic/spicy (onion, garlic, cumin and chilli), bitter (parsley, coriander), sour (lemon juice) and salt make up the flavour combination.

The dish probably originated in Egypt and spread through Arabic and Mediterranean countries, all characterised by their hot and dry climates. In these countries it is often served in a flat bread such as pitta with a green salad, an approach that rarely matches the colder, damper British climate. Even at the height of our summer! For this reason it is better to eat "British" falafel as recommended above.

Variations

Falafel is prepared and served in a wide variety of ways throughout the world. Some versions are distinctly spicy. Despite the fact that this is essentially a summer dish, if we want to eat it at other times of the year, we should employ the rule that the colder and damper our weather gets, the spicier that the falafel should be. Classic spices that can be used to achieve this are ground cumin and coriander seed, cayenne pepper and paprika.

Slow-roasted lamb shoulder with harissa, soy sauce, mustard and honey marinade

Ingredients

lamb shoulder
2 tbsp harissa sauce (this is a rough guide – spiciness
varies between different products)
1 tbsp soy sauce
1 tsp mustard
1 tbsp balsamic vinegar
1 tbsp honey
vegetables for steaming to serve

Method

Mix a paste of harissa, soy sauce, mustard, balsamic vinegar
and a dollop of honey. Smear this all over the lamb shoulder
and leave to marinade for an hour. Place in a roasting dish
on the middle shelf of the oven at around 140°C. Cook for
4 to 5 hours.

Serve it with plenty of steamed vegetables like broccoli,
asparagus, kale or chard. The leftovers make fantastic salad
ingredients. How about a lamb and pomegranate salad?

A classic winter warmer, this dish is great to put in the
oven on a Sunday morning before going out for a long walk
or some vigorous exercise, if you're that way inclined. The
smells are sensational and the meat is meltingly tender.

Harissa is a spicy North African sauce based on piri
piri: chilli peppers, tomatoes and paprika. Other ingredients vary depending on the brand and region of origin. It is
traditionally used as an appetiser and plays a crucial role in

this recipe as lamb is among the richest of meats. The other spicy ingredient, mustard, enhances this effect.

The sour flavour of the harissa and the vinegar also enhances digestibility by cutting through the lamb fat, while sweet honey nourishes friendly bacteria.

Variations

Overall, this is a very hot and rich dish and needs balancing if you struggle with very spicy food. This balance is best achieved with refreshing aromatic herbs like mint, chervil or coriander. You could also mix yoghurt with cucumber, a strategy that is only recommended with very spicy dishes as it does significantly slow motility. The lamb also combines well with bitter greens like rocket, dandelion or chicory.

Because this dish is more intense than the other recipes in this section, if you know that you have a weak stomach or are prone to IBS-type symptoms, it may be best to give it a miss.

Stuffed marrow

Serves 3

Ingredients

1 large marrow, peeled
100 g brown rice
2 tbsp olive oil
1 red onion, finely sliced
100 g chorizo, cut into small chunks
1 roasted red pepper, finely sliced ·
2 vine-ripened tomatoes, seeded and chopped
1 tbsp paprika
salt and freshly ground black pepper
(optional extras: beans, lentils, mushrooms, courgettes)

Method

Preheat the oven to 175°C. Partly cook the brown rice (about two-thirds cooked), then drain it.

Brown the onions and add the paprika, then the chorizo, which will release a nice red colour (the paprika within the chorizo).

After a minute or two, add the pepper (and beans/mushrooms/courgettes if you're using them).

After another couple of minutes, add the tomatoes, wait until the mixture is boiling again and then add the rice, which will soak up some of the moisture. Mix well.

Cut marrow in half lengthways, hollow out the seeds, leaving a decent amount of marrow as a base. Cut a thin flat strip out of the bottom marrow half – this helps to stop it rolling over. Put the marrow in the oven 10 minutes before the sauce is ready. Take marrow out and add the filling. Cook for about 15-20 minutes until piping hot and the marrow is just tender. To check if it is done, push the tip of a knife into the side, if it offers just a little resistance it is done. Serve with a dressed salad, spinach or other vegetables of choice.

This is a classic autumn dish. Warming and nourishing, it is ideal as the wind and rain blow in, and it is perfect for using up seasonal veggies. Simply spiced as it is with paprika, black pepper and chilli from the chorizo, it depends on olive oil and the sausage for its richness, a key requirement as the climate chills.

Variations

You can add chopped fresh aromatic herbs at the baking stage; basil, parsley, chives and oregano are all suitable.

Mellow spices, such as cumin and coriander, also complement it and are good additions in persistent damp weather.

"Add-ons"

Apple and tomato chutney

Makes 6 x 450 g pots

Ingredients

225 g red onions, peeled and chopped
1.8 kg tomatoes, peeled and chopped
225 g eating apples, peeled and chopped
650 g sugar
425 ml white malt vinegar
175 g sultanas
1 tbsp dairy salt
2 tsp ground ginger
3 tsp black pepper
3 tsp allspice
1 level tsp cayenne pepper
4 cloves garlic, finely chopped or crushed

Method

Put all the ingredients into a large stainless-steel pot. Bring
to the boil and simmer uncovered for around an hour. Pour
into sterilised jars.

One of the tricks with a condiment is to incorporate the
majority of the five flavours in the recipe, to an intense level,
thus stimulating and supporting all of the digestive functions and nourishing the general metabolism.

This is very much the result with this chutney, with sweet
(sultanas, apples, onions and sugar), sour (tomatoes, apples

271

and vinegar), salty/savoury (dairy salt) and spicy/pungent/ aromatic (onions, garlic, ginger, cayenne pepper, black pepper and allspice) all represented.

Variations

The only flavour that does not have a presence in the chutney is bitter. Bitter stimulates bowel movement so it is desirable in a condiment, particularly if you tend to be on the sluggish side. Try adding some turmeric or fenugreek or a few juniper berries to the mix for some bitterness.

In terms of the bulk of the chutney, bottling and preserving tends to be seasonal, using what's available rather than sticking rigidly to recipes. So, if you need to, you can swap the apples for pears or even for marrows. Or reduce the tomatoes by a third and add some chopped butternut squash.

Simple chicken broth

Ingredients

organic chicken carcass including the skin, or bones
from the butcher
1 stick celery, roughly chopped
1 carrot, roughly chopped
1 medium onion, roughly chopped
2 bay leaves
sprig of thyme
3 whole pepper corns
a couple of tomatoes or a tsp of apple cider vinegar (acid
  helps the bones break down, leaching the minerals into
  the broth)
3 sprigs parsley

Method

Get a cleaver out and smash up the bones. Put them in a big
saucepan with all other ingredients except the parsley, and
cover with water. If using more bones, add more water. Boil
the mixture over a high heat, then reduce to a simmer.

Using a large spoon, skim off any foam that appears on
top. This may continue for an hour. Continue to simmer for
3-6 hours, adding the parsley half an hour before comple-
tion. Strain the stock through a mesh sieve and cool as
quickly as possible before refrigerating. Skim off any fat too
that has developed on top.

Can be refrigerated for up to a week or frozen.

Bone stocks are quite simply the most nutritious, thrifty
and essential of all culinary creations. The bone marrow has

the nutrients that we need to make blood. The bones and skin have everything that we need to nourish skin, connective tissue and a whole lot of other structures in our bodies. And to top it all, many butchers are giving the bones away! They needn't cost a bean.

It comes as little surprise then that these stocks underpin just about every (non-vegetarian) cuisine in the world.

It seems odd now that the stock pot is no longer the hub of the modern kitchen. The reasons for this are probably twofold. The first, the rise of the supermarkets, has put a layer of cellophane between us and just about every food item that we buy. The second is that we are living in the era of cheap food: we now gorge on prime cuts.

In this recipe we have the "holy trinity" of stock veg; carrot, celery and onion. There is a logic to this classic combination, they give a rounded flavour profile – sweet (carrot), aromatic (onion) and bitter (celery). Add to this some sour (vinegar) and a few extra bitter and aromatic herbs to compensate for our damp climate and we have the ideal stock for Britain.

Variations

There is so much variety when it comes to stocks, especially when we look at the cuisines of other countries. These are definitely worth exploring.

Otherwise, the most important principle to employ when making a stock is to use up leftovers. Bones of course but also vegetable off-cuts, herb stalks, seasonal greens and medicinal tonic foods. All of these can combine to make us very healthy indeed.

Margot's tomato ketchup

Ingredients

5.5 kgs of tomatoes
1 kg onions
60 g garlic
30 g cloves
30 g ground fresh root ginger
170 g salt
½ tsp cayenne pepper
900 g sugar
1.2 litres apple cider vinegar

Method

Put all the ingredients except the sugar and vinegar into a big pot and boil slowly for two hours. Then pass through a blender, add the vinegar and sugar, bring to the boil and reduce to required thickness (the equivalent of thick cream). Pour into warm clean sterilised jars and seal.

This is such a delicious, delightfully balanced sauce that it has come to be known as "Liquid Gold" at home. Added to beans or any cooked meat, it is often the making of a meal. It contains a brilliant mix of spice, sour and sweet to stimulate appetite and digestion.

It's worth having a session once a year to make it, as you would with marmalade and pickles, and, if it's a bad year for blight, there's no shame in buying in the tomatoes fresh from the local market.

Spiced damson purée

Ingredients

2.5 kg damsons
600 g sugar
1.1 litres cider vinegar
12 whole cardamoms
60 g cloves
30 g cinnamon
15 g ground mace
15 g powdered ginger

Method

Stone the fruit, then put it in a bowl. If you have a food mill that will separate out the stones once the fruit is cooked, then you do not need to stone the damsons at this stage; just put them in a bowl. Put the rest of the ingredients in a pan and bring to the boil, then pour the mix over the fruit. Allow to sit for 24 hours.

Drain off the liquid and bring it back to the boil then pour it over the fruit again. Repeat this three times until the liquid is reduced and the fruit softened. Sieve the liquid and pass the fruit through a food mill. Return liquid and puréed fruit to the pan and reduce down to a thick liquid.

Bottle in hot sterilised jars and seal.

With its mix of sour, sweet and intense aromatics, this is the ideal accompaniment to fatty meat such as pork and liver. Sour cuts through the fat, while the aromatics stimulate motility to disperse it through the gut.

Variations

With very fatty food or a sluggish gut, more sourness is desirable. To achieve this, simply reduce the amount of sugar in the recipe. With very cold or damp weather you may want a spicier mix. In this case, add a little cayenne pepper.

Acknowledgements

It couldn't have been written without Lee Butler, Anna McGill, Dr Paul Watson, Charles and Tamsin Newington-Bridges.

At Short Books – Aurea Carpenter, Rebecca Nicolson, for patient editing Clemmie Jackson-Stops and more patient editing Elspeth Sinclair.

For sharing academic papers and info – Dr Paul Clayton, Dr Elaine Leong, Dr Judith Rowbotham, Prof. Richard Wrangham and Joanna Webber.

For teaching me – Steve Clavey, Prof. Zhang Ye, Dr Jia Yizhen, Shai Golan, Felicity Moir.

Also thanks to my clients, my mother, Dad, Lilli Cooper, Carry Dalq, Natasha Farrant, Bee Hayes, Liz at Sheepdrove, Henry McGrath, Gill McLay, Owen McNeir, Shara Routledge, Graham Symes, Jane Tatam, Dr Liz White and my old school and Oxford friends and family who saw me through the difficult years.

I'm a clinician rather than a chef and before writing this book recipes were largely alien to me, so I am grateful to my friend and gifted nutritional consultant Jamie Richards (www.jamierichards. co.uk) for providing a number of recipes for the book. If you are seeking further clarification regarding these recipes, however, the commentaries and variations sections are my own.

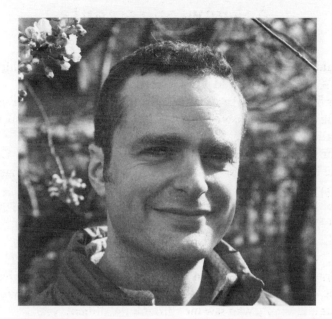

George Cooper studied biological sciences at Oxford
and during his studies developed a severe digestive
illness. After experiencing no benefit from conventional approaches to this illness, he looked increasingly
to Chinese medical techniques, and then embarked
on a long training in traditional Chinese medicine
at universities in the UK, China and Australia. He
now lives in Somerset and runs a busy clinic in Bristol
offering acupuncture, and advice on nutrition and
herbs. He also teaches regularly at the University of
Bristol Medical School and the College of Naturopathic
Medicine.

Index